RAMADAN MEDICATION GUIDE: SAFE AND EFFECTIVE DRUG USE WHILE FASTING

Abdool Samad (Sam) ILLAIEE
Healthcare Consultant Pharmacist

© 2024 Sam Illaiee

All rights reserved.

No part of this book may be reproduced, stored in a retrieval system, or transmitted in any form or by any means—electronic, mechanical, photocopying, recording, or otherwise—without prior written permission from the publisher, except in the case of brief quotations used in critical reviews or articles.

This book is intended for informational and educational purposes only. The author and publisher do not assume and hereby disclaim any liability to any party for any loss, damage, or disruption caused by errors or omissions, whether such errors or omissions result from negligence, accident, or any other cause.

Published by:
Sam ILLAIEE

For inquiries or permissions, bookings, coaching, mentoring and training contact Islandfarmacist@gmail.com

Cover design by: Sam ILLIAEE
First Edition

INTRODUCTION

The holy month of **Ramadan**, observed by millions of Muslims around the world, is a time for spiritual reflection, increased devotion, and self-discipline. One of the central practices of Ramadan is fasting from **dawn to sunset**, abstaining from food, drink, and other physical needs as a means of drawing closer to God. While fasting is a profound spiritual practice, it also presents unique challenges for individuals who rely on medications for managing chronic conditions or acute health issues.

For those on regular medication, maintaining therapeutic effectiveness while adhering to the fasting schedule requires careful planning and adjustment. Medications may need to be taken at different times or in different dosages to avoid interfering with the fast, ensure proper absorption, and minimize side effects such as dehydration, fatigue, or nausea. Importantly, the timing of doses, the type of medication, and the condition being treated all influence how a patient's medication regimen should be modified during Ramadan.

This guide aims to provide **comprehensive recommendations** for managing medications during Ramadan, offering insights for both healthcare providers and patients. It covers a wide array of medication categories, from common chronic disease treatments like insulin and antihypertensives, to specialized therapies used in cancer treatment and palliative care. Whether the patient is managing diabetes, hypertension, cancer, mental health conditions, or other medical needs, this guide is intended to help healthcare providers and patients make informed decisions about how to adjust medication regimens during Ramadan.

Key Considerations for Medication Use During Ramadan:

- **Medication Timing**: Many medications need to be taken at specific times to be effective. For patients observing the fast, adjustments may be necessary to ensure that medication is taken during non-fasting hours (i.e., after Iftar or before Suhoor).
- **Hydration**: Some medications may have side effects that are compounded by dehydration, which is common during fasting. Ensuring adequate hydration during non-fasting hours is essential.
- **Therapeutic Effectiveness**: Ensuring that the medications continue to work effectively throughout the fasting period without causing harm to the patient is paramount. Adjusting dosages or switching medications may be necessary to maintain efficacy.
- **Patient Safety**: Patient safety is the primary concern. Special attention should be paid to high-risk patients, including those with chronic conditions, the elderly, pregnant women, and those on complex regimens.

Stay Updated and Seek Medical Advice:

It is important to note that the advice provided in this guide is meant to offer general recommendations. Medication practices, dosing, and fasting-related adjustments can vary widely based on individual circumstances. As such, it is **essential for patients to consult with their healthcare provider** before making any changes to their medication regimen. Medical advice should be based on up-to-date, individualized assessments, as treatment protocols may evolve over time and vary depending on the region and healthcare guidelines.

By utilizing this guide, patients and healthcare providers can ensure that Ramadan fasting does not interfere with health management, while also preserving the spiritual benefits of this important month.

CHAPTER 1: CARDIOVASCULAR MEDICATIONS

Managing cardiovascular health during Ramadan is critical, especially for individuals with hypertension, heart disease, or arrhythmias. Fasting affects the timing of medication administration, which can impact drug efficacy and side effects. This chapter provides guidelines for managing cardiovascular medications, emphasizing timing adjustments to maintain both health and religious practices.

Beta-Blockers

Beta-blockers are commonly prescribed to manage conditions like hypertension, heart failure, and arrhythmias. These medications work by reducing the heart rate and blood pressure, which can be affected by fasting. To optimize their effectiveness during Ramadan, it is crucial to adjust the timing of beta-blocker doses.

Drug Name	Timing Recommendation	Notes
Bisoprolol	After Iftar and before or	Take with food

	with Suhoor	to avoid stomach irritation.
Metoprolol	After Iftar and before or with Suhoor	Monitor for dizziness and fatigue, especially when transitioning from sitting or standing.
Atenolol	After Iftar and before or with Suhoor	Ensure adequate hydration to avoid dehydration-related side effects.

General Advice for Beta-Blockers:
- Beta-blockers should be taken consistently at the same time each day, even during Ramadan.
- Monitor for side effects such as dizziness, especially when standing up, as beta-blockers can lower blood pressure.

ACE Inhibitors and Angiotensin Receptor Blockers (ARBs)

ACE inhibitors and ARBs are key in managing hypertension, heart failure, and chronic kidney disease. During Ramadan, patients on these medications should adjust their dosing schedules to avoid complications like dehydration or hypotension.

Drug Name	Timing Recommendation	Notes
Lisinopril	After Iftar and before or with Suhoor	Monitor for dizziness and low blood pressure, particularly at the beginning of Ramadan.

Enalapril	After Iftar and before or with Suhoor	May cause a drop in blood pressure, so ensure appropriate hydration.
Valsartan	After Iftar and before or with Suhoor	Adjust timing if taking multiple antihypertensives to avoid interactions.

General Advice for ACE Inhibitors and ARBs:

- These medications should be taken after Iftar or before or with Suhoor, as they may lower blood pressure, leading to symptoms like dizziness, especially during fasting hours.
- Ensure patients are monitoring their blood pressure regularly and adjusting hydration during non-fasting hours.

Calcium Channel Blockers (CCBs)

CCBs are often used to treat hypertension, angina, and arrhythmias. They help relax and widen blood vessels, improving blood flow. As fasting can cause dehydration and electrolyte imbalance, timing adjustments are needed to minimize these risks.

Drug Name	Timing Recommendation	Notes
Amlodipine	After Iftar and before or with Suhoor	Can cause swelling in the lower extremities; monitor for signs of fluid retention.
Nifedipine	After Iftar and before or with Suhoor	Ensure regular monitoring of heart rate and blood

		pressure, as CCBs can cause both hypotension and bradycardia.

General Advice for CCBs:

- These medications should be taken after Iftar and before or with Suhoor to avoid fluctuations in blood pressure and ensure consistent efficacy.
- Hydration is essential, as dehydration can enhance the risk of adverse effects like hypotension.

General Tips for Managing Cardiovascular Medications During Ramadan

1. **Hydration**: Proper hydration during non-fasting hours is essential for patients on cardiovascular medications, particularly beta-blockers, ACE inhibitors, ARBs, and CCBs. Dehydration can exacerbate side effects like dizziness, fatigue, and hypotension.
2. **Consistent Timing**: Patients should take their medications consistently at the same time each day. Modifying the timing to after Iftar and before or with Suhoor helps maintain the medication's effectiveness while accommodating fasting hours.
3. **Monitoring**: Regular monitoring of blood pressure and heart rate is recommended, especially for those on medications that affect cardiovascular function. Encourage patients to check for symptoms such as dizziness, excessive fatigue, or heart palpitations.
4. **Diet**: Advise patients to avoid large, heavy meals at Iftar and Suhoor, which can further lower blood pressure and make side effects worse. A balanced meal is ideal for maintaining stable blood pressure levels.

CHAPTER 2: ANTIDIABETICS

Managing diabetes during Ramadan requires careful planning to avoid both hypoglycemia (low blood sugar) and hyperglycemia (high blood sugar). Fasting, along with the restriction of food and drink, can impact the way insulin and oral diabetes medications work. The goal is to adjust medication regimens to ensure optimal blood sugar control while maintaining the safety of the patient during fasting hours.

Insulin Therapy

For individuals on insulin therapy, careful adjustments are necessary due to the long hours of fasting and the potential for changes in insulin sensitivity. Here are the recommended adjustments for various types of insulin:

Type of Insulin	Timing Recommendation	Notes
Long-acting (e.g., Glargine)	After Iftar and before or with Suhoor	Reduce the dose by 25–50% based on pre-fasting blood glucose levels.
Intermediate-acting (e.g., NPH)	After Iftar and before or with Suhoor	Split doses if necessary to adjust for fasting.
Rapid-acting (e.g., Lispro)	After Iftar and before or with Suhoor	Adjust based on carbohydrate intake at Iftar and Suhoor.
Premixed Insulin (e.g., Humalog Mix)	After Iftar and before or with Suhoor	Adjust doses for pre-dawn and evening

| | | doses to prevent hypoglycemia. |

General Advice for Insulin Therapy:

- **Monitoring**: Patients should monitor blood glucose levels frequently during Ramadan—especially before Suhoor, before Iftar, and at two hours after Iftar. This will help adjust insulin doses as needed.
- **Avoiding Hypoglycemia**: Reduce insulin doses at Suhoor (particularly for long-acting or premixed insulin) to prevent hypoglycemia, especially for patients who are well-controlled.
- **Break the Fast if Necessary**: Patients should break the fast if their blood glucose falls below 3.3 mmol/L or exceeds 16.6 mmol/L, or if symptoms of hypoglycemia or hyperglycemia occur.

Oral Antidiabetic Medications

For individuals on oral diabetes medications, the goal is to adjust doses to prevent hypoglycemia and ensure proper glucose control during the fasting period. Here are the recommendations for common oral antidiabetic medications:

Drug Name	Timing Recommendation	Notes
Metformin (Immediate-release)	After Iftar and before or with Suhoor	Continue regular dosing, but avoid taking at Suhoor if possible to reduce gastrointestinal

		side effects.
Metformin (Extended-release)	After Iftar and before or with Suhoor	Split doses if prescribed BID; ensure regular blood sugar monitoring.
Sulfonylureas (e.g., Gliclazide)	After Iftar and before or with Suhoor	Reduce Suhoor dose to avoid hypoglycemia, especially in elderly patients.
SGLT-2 Inhibitors (e.g., Dapagliflozin)	After Iftar and before or with Suhoor	Caution for dehydration due to fasting; monitor renal function and fluid status.
Thiazolidinediones (e.g., Pioglitazone)	After Iftar and before or with Suhoor	May cause fluid retention; monitor for swelling.
GLP-1 Receptor Agonists (e.g., Liraglutide)	After Iftar and before or with Suhoor	Can reduce appetite; patients should monitor for any signs of nausea.

General Advice for Oral Antidiabetics:

- **Monitoring**: Regular monitoring of blood glucose is crucial, especially for patients on sulfonylureas, as these can cause hypoglycemia if doses are not adjusted properly.
- **Hydration**: Encourage patients to stay hydrated during non-fasting hours, particularly those on SGLT-2 inhibitors, as dehydration can increase the risk of side effects.
- **Adjusting Doses**: Sulfonylureas should be reduced at Suhoor, especially if good glucose control is achieved. For metformin, it is typically safe to continue the usual dose, but the patient should be mindful of symptoms such as stomach discomfort.

Managing Blood Glucose Levels

Fasting during Ramadan can significantly alter blood glucose control, making it essential for diabetic patients to monitor their blood sugar levels frequently. The following are key times for blood glucose monitoring:

1. **Before Suhoor**: To check baseline glucose before fasting.
2. **Mid-morning (around 10 a.m.)**: To check for fluctuations in glucose levels.
3. **Before Iftar**: To measure glucose before breaking the fast.
4. **Two hours after Iftar**: To check for postprandial (after meal) glucose spikes.
5. **Before bedtime**: To ensure glucose levels stabilize before sleep.

Blood Glucose Targets During Ramadan

- **Before Suhoor**: Ideally between **4–7 mmol/L**.
- **Before Iftar**: Ideally between **4–7 mmol/L**.
- **Post-Iftar (2 hours)**: Ideally less than **10 mmol/L**.

Recommendations for Specific Patient Groups

Patients with Poorly Controlled Diabetes

- These patients should ideally avoid fasting, as they may experience frequent fluctuations in blood glucose that could lead to complications such as ketoacidosis or severe hypoglycemia.
- In cases where fasting is non-negotiable, stricter blood glucose monitoring is essential, and medication doses should be adjusted to prevent hypoglycemia.

Elderly Patients

- Older individuals on oral medications or insulin are at higher risk for hypoglycemia due to potential changes in renal function and the body's response to fasting.
- Adjust doses of sulfonylureas and insulin carefully, and monitor blood glucose more frequently.

Key Takeaways for Antidiabetics During Ramadan:

- **Pre-Ramadan Assessment**: Patients should meet with

their healthcare provider before Ramadan to review their medication regimen and make adjustments if necessary.
- **Hydration**: Ensure patients drink plenty of water during non-fasting hours to avoid dehydration, particularly those on SGLT-2 inhibitors or diuretics.
- **Blood Glucose Monitoring**: Regular monitoring is essential to ensure blood sugar levels stay within a safe range during fasting hours.
- **Break the Fast if Necessary**: Advise patients to break the fast if blood glucose falls below 3.3 mmol/L or rises above 16.6 mmol/L, or if they experience symptoms of hypoglycemia or hyperglycemia.

CHAPTER 3: ANTIBIOTICS

Antibiotics are commonly prescribed for infections, and managing them during Ramadan requires adjusting the timing of doses to align with fasting hours. The goal is to ensure the effectiveness of the antibiotic regimen while minimizing side effects and avoiding interactions with food or hydration during fasting.

General Considerations for Antibiotic Use During Ramadan

- **Timing**: Antibiotics should generally be taken **after Iftar and before or with Suhoor** to avoid interfering with fasting hours. This allows the patient to take their full dose after breaking the fast and helps prevent gastrointestinal irritation.
- **Hydration**: Adequate hydration is crucial during Ramadan, especially for patients on antibiotics that can cause dehydration or affect kidney function.
- **Completing the Course**: Patients must complete the full course of antibiotics as prescribed, even if they feel better before the course is finished. Skipping doses or stopping treatment early can lead to antibiotic resistance and treatment failure.

Commonly Used Antibiotics and Timing Adjustments

Drug Name	Timing Recommendation	Notes
Amoxicillin	After Iftar and before or with Suhoor	Ensure doses are evenly spaced if taking multiple doses daily.
Augmentin	After Iftar and before or with Suhoor	Take with food to avoid stomach upset.
Azithromycin	After Iftar (OD for 3–5 days)	Short courses; space doses if needed.
Ciprofloxacin	After Iftar and before or with Suhoor	Avoid taking with dairy or calcium-rich products, as they can interfere with absorption.
Doxycycline	After Iftar	Take with a full glass of water and avoid lying down immediately to prevent esophageal irritation.
Clarithromycin	After Iftar and before or with Suhoor	Ensure hydration to avoid side effects like dizziness.
Levofloxacin	After Iftar and before or with Suhoor	Take with food if needed to reduce nausea.

General Advice for Antibiotics:

- **Adherence to Dosing Schedule**: It's essential that patients take their antibiotics at the correct intervals to maintain therapeutic drug levels in the bloodstream. Taking antibiotics after Iftar and before or with Suhoor helps align with fasting hours and ensures better absorption.
- **Gastrointestinal Upset**: Many antibiotics, particularly those in the penicillin and cephalosporin classes, can cause

gastrointestinal distress. Taking these medications with food or water after Iftar and before or with Suhoor can help reduce side effects like nausea, diarrhea, and stomach cramps.
- **Hydration**: Patients should be encouraged to drink plenty of water during non-fasting hours, especially when taking antibiotics that can increase the risk of dehydration (e.g., diuretics or certain antibiotics like trimethoprim-sulfamethoxazole).

Managing Antibiotics for Specific Infections

Upper Respiratory Tract Infections (URTIs)

For mild upper respiratory tract infections, antibiotics like amoxicillin or azithromycin may be prescribed. The timing of these medications ensures effectiveness while avoiding side effects.

Recommended Antibiotic	Timing Recommendation	Notes
Amoxicillin (250–500 mg)	After Iftar and before or with Suhoor	Continue for the full course.
Azithromycin (250–500 mg)	After Iftar (OD for 3–5 days)	A single dose daily for 3-5 days.

Lower Respiratory Tract Infections (LRTIs)

For bacterial pneumonia or other lower respiratory infections, antibiotics like Augmentin or ciprofloxacin are often used. Ensure the patient completes the entire course of antibiotics.

Recommended Antibiotic	Timing Recommendation	Notes
Augmentin (1 g)	After Iftar and before or with Suhoor	Space doses evenly if taking BID.
Levofloxacin (250–500 mg)	After Iftar and before or with Suhoor	Monitor hydration to prevent dehydration.

Urinary Tract Infections (UTIs)

For UTIs, common antibiotics like nitrofurantoin or ciprofloxacin are prescribed. Timing should be adjusted to minimize side effects and ensure effective treatment.

Recommended Antibiotic	Timing Recommendation	Notes
Nitrofurantoin (Immediate-release)	After Iftar and before or with Suhoor	Ensure hydration to prevent kidney issues.
Ciprofloxacin (250–500 mg)	After Iftar and before or with Suhoor	Take with water; avoid antacids or dairy.

Common Antibiotics and Their Timing Adjustments

Penicillins

Penicillins are commonly used to treat a variety of bacterial infections, including streptococcal throat infections and UTIs. These antibiotics are generally well-tolerated but may cause gastrointestinal upset, particularly if taken on an empty stomach.

Drug Name	Timing Recommendation	Notes
Amoxicillin	After Iftar and before or with Suhoor	Can be taken with or without food; take with food if GI upset occurs.
Augmentin (Amoxicillin + Clavulanic Acid)	After Iftar and before or with Suhoor	Take with food to reduce stomach upset and improve absorption.

General Advice for Penicillins:

- **Food Interaction**: Some penicillins, such as Augmentin, should be taken with food to reduce gastrointestinal side effects.
- **Hydration**: Encourage adequate hydration between

Iftar and Suhoor, especially for patients on antibiotics like amoxicillin, which can be excreted through the kidneys.

Cephalosporins

Cephalosporins are a class of antibiotics used to treat a wide variety of infections, including respiratory, skin, and urinary tract infections. These medications may cause gastrointestinal disturbances, so taking them with food is recommended.

Drug Name	Timing Recommendation	Notes
Cefuroxime	After Iftar and before or with Suhoor	Take with food to avoid stomach upset.
Cefalexin	After Iftar and before or with Suhoor	Can be taken with food to improve absorption.

General Advice for Cephalosporins:

- **Food Interaction**: To minimize gastrointestinal upset, take cephalosporins like cefuroxime and cefalexin **after Iftar and before or with Suhoor.**
- **Hydration**: Ensure proper hydration to avoid kidney issues, as cephalosporins are eliminated through the kidneys.

Fluoroquinolones

Fluoroquinolones are broad-spectrum antibiotics used to treat a range of bacterial infections, including UTIs, respiratory infections, and gastrointestinal infections. They should be taken with food to reduce gastrointestinal side effects, but should not be taken with dairy products, as calcium can interfere with their absorption.

Drug Name	Timing Recommendation	Notes
Ciprofloxacin	After Iftar and before or	Avoid taking with

	with Suhoor	dairy or calcium-rich foods.
Levofloxacin	After Iftar and before or with Suhoor	Ensure proper hydration to avoid potential kidney issues.

General Advice for Fluoroquinolones:

- **Food and Drug Interactions**: Avoid taking fluoroquinolones with dairy, antacids, or calcium supplements, as these can reduce absorption.
- **Hydration**: Fluoroquinolones can increase the risk of kidney toxicity, so maintaining adequate hydration is crucial.

Macrolides

Macrolides, such as azithromycin and clarithromycin, are commonly prescribed for respiratory and skin infections. They should generally be taken after meals to avoid gastrointestinal upset and enhance absorption.

Drug Name	Timing Recommendation	Notes
Azithromycin	After Iftar and before or with Suhoor	Take with food to reduce gastrointestinal side effects.
Clarithromycin	After Iftar and before or with Suhoor	Take with food to avoid GI discomfort.

General Advice for Macrolides:

- **Food Interaction**: Take macrolides with food to minimize gastrointestinal upset and ensure proper absorption.
- **Hydration**: Ensure that patients drink plenty of fluids between Iftar and Suhoor to avoid dehydration and maintain kidney function.

Tetracyclines

Tetracyclines, such as doxycycline, are commonly used to treat infections caused by bacteria, including acne, respiratory infections, and STDs. They should not be taken with dairy products, calcium, or antacids, as these can impair absorption.

Drug Name	Timing Recommendation	Notes
Doxycycline	After Iftar and before or with Suhoor	Take with water; avoid lying down immediately after taking to prevent esophageal irritation.

General Advice for Tetracyclines:

- **Food and Drug Interactions**: Avoid taking tetracyclines with dairy, antacids, or calcium-rich foods to ensure proper absorption.
- **Hydration**: Drink a full glass of water when taking doxycycline to avoid esophageal irritation.

Special Considerations for Antibiotic Use in Ramadan

Elderly Patients

- Elderly patients are at increased risk for side effects due to altered drug metabolism and kidney function. Ensure antibiotics are dosed appropriately, with adjustments made for renal function when necessary.
- For those who are more susceptible to dehydration or electrolyte imbalances, special attention should be given to drugs like diuretics or those that may affect renal function.

Children

- Children may experience dehydration more quickly, especially if they are on antibiotics that increase fluid loss. Pediatric dosing should be carefully considered, with

adjustments to avoid excessive dosing during fasting hours.
- Always ensure that children take their full course of antibiotics, even if they seem to recover before the end of treatment.

Pregnancy and Breastfeeding
- Pregnant and breastfeeding women who require antibiotics should consult their healthcare provider to ensure the safety of both the mother and the baby. Some antibiotics, like tetracyclines, are contraindicated during pregnancy due to the risk of harming fetal development.

Adherence
- Adherence to the prescribed course of antibiotics is crucial to prevent resistance and ensure the infection is fully treated. Patients should be reminded not to skip doses and to complete the full course of treatment, even if they start feeling better.

Key Takeaways for Antibiotics During Ramadan:

- **Timing**: Take antibiotics **after Iftar and before or with Suhoor** to align with fasting hours. This ensures better absorption and minimizes gastrointestinal side effects.
- **Hydration**: Drink plenty of water during non-fasting hours to prevent dehydration, especially for antibiotics that can cause kidney issues.
- **Completing the Course**: It is critical that patients complete their full course of antibiotics to prevent antibiotic resistance and ensure the infection is fully treated.
- **Adherence**: Encourage patients to adhere strictly to the prescribed dosing schedule and monitor for any potential side effects, including gastrointestinal disturbances.

CHAPTER 4: PAIN MANAGEMENT AND ANALGESICS

Pain management during Ramadan requires careful attention to medication schedules, particularly since fasting means avoiding food and drink during the day. The goal is to provide adequate pain relief while minimizing the risk of side effects, especially those related to dehydration or gastrointestinal irritation. This chapter covers the use of analgesics, including non-steroidal anti-inflammatory drugs (NSAIDs), opioids, and other pain-relieving medications, with a focus on optimizing their use during fasting hours.

Non-Steroidal Anti-Inflammatory Drugs (NSAIDs)

NSAIDs are commonly used to manage pain, inflammation, and fever. However, they can cause gastrointestinal irritation, especially when taken on an empty stomach, and may increase the risk of dehydration during fasting. It is crucial to adjust the timing of these medications during Ramadan to minimize side effects.

Drug Name	Timing Recommendation	Notes
Paracetamol	After Iftar and before or with Suhoor	Generally well-tolerated, hydrate well to avoid dehydration.

Ibuprofen	After Iftar and before or with Suhoor	Take with food to minimize gastric irritation.
Diclofenac	After Iftar and before or with Suhoor	Take with food to prevent gastrointestinal upset.
Celecoxib	After Iftar and before or with Suhoor	Preferable for long-term use in patients at risk of GI issues.
Mefenamic Acid	After Iftar and before or with Suhoor	Take with food to prevent stomach discomfort.

General Advice for NSAIDs:

- **Food Intake**: To avoid gastrointestinal irritation, NSAIDs should be taken after Iftar and before or with Suhoor, ideally with food.
- **Hydration**: NSAIDs can increase the risk of kidney issues, particularly if dehydration occurs. Ensure adequate hydration between Iftar and Suhoor.
- **Duration of Use**: Limit the duration of NSAID use during Ramadan, especially in patients with a history of gastrointestinal problems, kidney disease, or heart failure.

Opioids for Severe Pain

Opioid analgesics are used for managing severe pain, such as post-surgical pain or pain from injuries. Since opioids can cause drowsiness, constipation, and respiratory depression, they must be used cautiously during Ramadan, particularly when adjusting timing and dosage to avoid side effects that may disrupt fasting.

Drug Name	Timing Recommendation	Notes
Tramadol	After Iftar and before or with Suhoor	Use lowest effective dose; monitor for dizziness and sedation.

Morphine (Extended Release)	After Iftar and before or with Suhoor	Adjust doses gradually to avoid withdrawal symptoms.
Codeine	After Iftar and before or with Suhoor	Monitor for drowsiness, avoid operating heavy machinery.

General Advice for Opioids:

- **Monitoring**: Patients should be closely monitored for side effects like drowsiness, dizziness, and respiratory depression.
- **Hydration**: Opioids can cause constipation, which may be aggravated by dehydration. Ensure adequate fluid intake during non-fasting hours.
- **Avoiding Drowsiness**: Since opioids may cause sedation, it is advisable to take these medications after Iftar and before or with Suhoor to ensure patients have time to rest and recover.

Alternative Analgesics

For patients who are unable to tolerate NSAIDs or opioids, alternative analgesics like acetaminophen (paracetamol) may be recommended. These medications are generally safer for long-term use but should still be used with caution, especially in patients with liver or kidney problems.

Drug Name	Timing Recommendation	Notes
Paracetamol (Acetaminophen)	After Iftar and before or with Suhoor	Generally safe when taken at recommended doses. Avoid exceeding the maximum daily dose.

General Advice for Alternative Analgesics:

- **Liver Function**: Patients with liver disease should limit their use of acetaminophen to avoid liver toxicity.

- **Hydration**: Ensure adequate hydration as paracetamol may increase the risk of liver damage when dehydration occurs.

Steroids (Corticosteroids)

Steroids such as **dexamethasone** and **prednisone** are used in inflamatory treatment to reduce inflammation, treat side effects of chemotherapy, and manage certain types of cancer like lymphoma or leukemia. Steroids also help improve appetite and mood.

Considerations During Ramadan:

- **Timing**: Steroids are often taken in the morning to mimic the body's natural cortisol cycle. If taken in high doses or for prolonged periods, it is essential to ensure they are taken **after Iftar** and **before Suhoor** to minimize the impact on fasting.
- **Side Effects**: Steroids can cause increased appetite, fluid retention, and mood swings, which could affect patients during fasting hours. Managing the timing and dose during Ramadan can help mitigate some of these issues.

Topical Analgesics

Topical analgesics, such as creams and patches, can provide localized pain relief without systemic effects. These are particularly useful for musculoskeletal pain or minor injuries. These medications can be used during fasting without affecting the fast itself, but timing considerations for hydration and overall comfort should still be considered.

Drug Name	Timing Recommendation	Notes
Topical Diclofenac Gel	After Iftar and before or with Suhoor, but anytime	Use as directed on the affected area; avoid broken skin.

| Lidocaine Patches | After Iftar and before or with Suhoor, but anytime | For localized pain relief; effective for muscle or joint pain. |

General Advice for Topical Analgesics:

- **Application**: Apply only to intact skin and avoid use near mucous membranes (mouth, eyes).
- **Monitoring**: Observe for skin reactions or irritation after application.

Managing Chronic Pain During Ramadan

For individuals with chronic pain conditions, such as arthritis or back pain, adjusting pain medication schedules during Ramadan can help maintain both effective pain control and fasting compliance. Here are some strategies for managing chronic pain:

1. **Adjust Doses for Fasting Hours**: Long-acting medications can be taken after Iftar, while shorter-acting medications may be used during Suhoor to prevent breakthrough pain.
2. **Non-Pharmacologic Methods**: Encourage the use of heat or cold packs, physical therapy, and other non-pharmacologic interventions to manage pain without medication.
3. **Monitor for Side Effects**: Ensure that patients are not experiencing excessive pain or adverse effects such as dizziness, nausea, or dehydration due to their medication regimen.

Key Takeaways for Pain Management During Ramadan:

1. **Timing**: For most pain medications, take **after Iftar and before or with Suhoor** to avoid disrupting fasting. This

allows for proper absorption and minimizes side effects.
2. **Hydration**: Ensure adequate fluid intake between Iftar and Suhoor to prevent dehydration, which can exacerbate side effects such as kidney issues or gastrointestinal discomfort.
3. **Medication Selection**: NSAIDs are effective for mild to moderate pain but should be used cautiously in patients with gastrointestinal issues or kidney disease. For severe pain, opioids should be used at the lowest effective dose, with careful monitoring for sedation and other side effects.
4. **Monitoring**: Regular monitoring of pain levels, medication side effects, and overall hydration status is essential to ensure safe and effective pain management during Ramadan.

CHAPTER 5: GASTROINTESTINAL (GI) DRUGS

Managing gastrointestinal conditions during Ramadan requires careful consideration of medication schedules to minimize side effects while ensuring effective treatment. During fasting, patients with conditions like acid reflux, constipation, diarrhea, IBS, and Crohn's disease must adjust their medication regimen to maintain proper digestive health while respecting fasting practices.

Proton Pump Inhibitors (PPIs) and H2 Receptor Antagonists

PPIs are commonly prescribed to treat conditions like gastroesophageal reflux disease (GERD) and peptic ulcers. These medications work by reducing stomach acid production and can help prevent acid reflux symptoms during fasting. Timing adjustments are necessary to prevent symptoms like heartburn and to optimize drug efficacy.

Drug Name	Timing Recommendation	Notes
Omeprazole	After Iftar and before or	Best taken on an empty

	with Suhoor	stomach; avoid food for 30 minutes after taking it.
Esomeprazole	After Iftar and before or with Suhoor	Avoid combining with antacids immediately.
Pantoprazole	After Iftar and before or with Suhoor	Take 30 minutes before Suhoor for optimal effect.
Lansoprazole	After Iftar and before or with Suhoor	Ensure a 30-minute window before eating.
Ranitidine	After Iftar and before or with Suhoor	H2 blockers can be effective for acid reflux during fasting hours.

General Advice for PPIs and H2 Receptor Antagonists:

- **Timing**: These medications should be taken **after Iftar and before or with Suhoor** to help manage acid levels and prevent heartburn during fasting hours.
- **Food Interaction**: PPIs should be taken on an empty stomach before eating for optimal absorption. Antacids should be avoided immediately before or after taking PPIs, as they can interfere with the medication's effectiveness.

Constipation Management

Constipation is a common issue during Ramadan due to changes in diet and reduced water intake. Managing constipation effectively is essential to prevent discomfort and maintain regular bowel movements. Several medications can be used to treat constipation while fasting.

Drug Name	Timing Recommendation	Notes
Lactulose	After Iftar and before or with Suhoor	Ensure adequate hydration to avoid dehydration.

Polyethylene Glycol (PEG)	After Iftar and before or with Suhoor	Space doses at least 8 hours apart if taking BID.
Bisacodyl	After Iftar	Use short-term for relief; avoid long-term use to prevent dependency.
Psyllium	After Iftar and before or with Suhoor	Take with plenty of water to prevent bloating and gas.

General Advice for Constipation Medications:

- **Hydration**: Increased water intake is crucial to alleviate constipation. Patients should drink plenty of water between Iftar and Suhoor.
- **Fiber**: Encourage a diet high in fiber, which can naturally alleviate constipation. Fiber supplements, such as psyllium, can help but require plenty of water to avoid worsening symptoms.
- **Short-Term Use**: Laxatives like bisacodyl should only be used for short-term relief to avoid dependency.

Diarrhea Management

Diarrhea can be triggered by dietary changes during Ramadan, such as the consumption of fried foods or spicy meals at Iftar. It is important to manage diarrhea effectively to avoid dehydration and other complications.

Drug Name	Timing Recommendation	Notes
Loperamide	After Iftar and before or with Suhoor	Take as needed for acute diarrhea; do not exceed recommended dose.
Racecadotril	After Iftar and before or with Suhoor	Reduces water secretion in the intestine and can help

		manage diarrhea.
Oral Rehydration Salts (ORS)	After Iftar and before or with Suhoor	Replenish lost fluids and electrolytes; space doses appropriately.

General Advice for Diarrhea Medications:

- **Rehydration**: Oral rehydration salts (ORS) are essential for preventing dehydration. They should be taken regularly to restore fluid and electrolyte balance.
- **Hydration**: Ensure that the patient drinks plenty of fluids between Iftar and Suhoor, especially if diarrhea occurs during fasting hours.
- **Avoiding Dehydration**: Loperamide can be used to control acute diarrhea, but it should be used cautiously to avoid exacerbating dehydration.

Irritable Bowel Syndrome (IBS) and Other Functional GI Disorders

IBS is a chronic condition that can cause symptoms like abdominal pain, bloating, and irregular bowel movements. Managing IBS during Ramadan can be challenging due to dietary changes, stress, and changes in meal timing. Medications can help manage IBS symptoms, allowing patients to maintain a normal fasting schedule.

Drug Name	Timing Recommendation	Notes
Mebeverine	After Iftar and before or with Suhoor	An antispasmodic that helps reduce abdominal pain and cramping.
Peppermint Oil Capsules	After Iftar and before or with Suhoor	Can help relieve bloating and discomfort.
Hyoscine Butylbromide	After Iftar and before or with Suhoor	Useful for reducing spasm-related pain and discomfort.

General Advice for IBS Management:
- **Diet**: Avoid foods that may trigger IBS symptoms, such as fatty or spicy foods, during Iftar and Suhoor.
- **Stress Management**: Stress can exacerbate IBS symptoms, so incorporating relaxation techniques such as deep breathing or mindfulness during fasting hours may help.
- **Fiber Intake**: A high-fiber diet can help regulate bowel movements, so encourage the consumption of fiber-rich foods during non-fasting hours.

Crohn's Disease and Ulcerative Colitis (Inflammatory Bowel Diseases)

For patients with inflammatory bowel diseases (IBD) like Crohn's disease and ulcerative colitis, it is important to adjust medications to prevent flare-ups and manage symptoms like abdominal pain, diarrhea, and inflammation. The timing of medications plays a crucial role in managing these conditions while fasting.

Drug Name	Timing Recommendation	Notes
Mesalazine	After Iftar and before or with Suhoor	Continue for the full course to prevent flare-ups.
Sulfasalazine	After Iftar and before or with Suhoor	Space doses as prescribed, with adequate hydration.
Biologic Agents (e.g., Adalimumab)	After Iftar and before or with Suhoor	Administer according to the prescribed schedule.

General Advice for IBD Medications:
- **Medication Adherence**: Ensure patients complete the full course of medications, even during Ramadan, to avoid disease flare-ups.
- **Dietary Adjustments**: Avoid foods that trigger

inflammation or irritation, such as spicy foods, dairy, and high-fiber foods during Iftar and Suhoor.
- **Hydration**: Staying hydrated is crucial, especially for patients on medications like sulfasalazine, which can affect kidney function.

Antiemetics (Anti-Nausea Drugs)

Cancer treatments, particularly chemotherapy, are known to cause nausea and vomiting. Antiemetics are crucial for managing these side effects and improving the quality of life for cancer patients.

- **5-HT3 Receptor Antagonists (e.g., Ondansetron, Granisetron)**: These drugs block serotonin, which can trigger nausea and vomiting after chemotherapy.
- **NK1 Receptor Antagonists (e.g., Aprepitant)**: Used in combination with other antiemetics to control nausea associated with chemotherapy.
- **Corticosteroids (e.g., Dexamethasone)**: Often used as part of the antiemetic regimen to reduce nausea and inflammation.

Considerations During Ramadan:

- **Timing**: These medications are typically taken before or after chemotherapy sessions. It may be necessary to adjust dosing times to align with **after Iftar** and **before Suhoor**, especially when managing nausea during fasting.
- **Hydration**: Some antiemetics, especially corticosteroids, can cause fluid retention and dehydration. It's important to monitor fluid intake during non-fasting hours to manage side effects effectively.

Key Takeaways for GI Medications During Ramadan:

1. **Timing**: Most GI medications, including PPIs, laxatives,

antispasmodics, and IBD medications, should be taken **after Iftar and before or with Suhoor** to ensure effectiveness and minimize side effects.
2. **Hydration**: Adequate hydration is essential for managing constipation, diarrhea, and other GI disorders. Patients should drink plenty of fluids between Iftar and Suhoor.
3. **Dietary Adjustments**: Advise patients to avoid triggering foods, such as spicy or fatty meals, during fasting hours. Fiber-rich foods can help manage constipation and IBS symptoms.
4. **Medication Adherence**: Patients should complete their full course of medications as prescribed, especially for chronic conditions like IBD, to prevent flare-ups.

CHAPTER 6: EPILEPSY AND ANTICONVULSANTS

Epilepsy is a neurological condition that can be managed effectively with anticonvulsant medications. However, fasting during Ramadan can present challenges for individuals with epilepsy, particularly with regard to medication timing and the potential risk of seizures. Adjustments to the timing and dosage of anticonvulsants are necessary to ensure that individuals maintain seizure control while observing their fast.

General Considerations for Epilepsy Medications

- **Timing**: Most anticonvulsants should be taken **after Iftar and before or with Suhoor** to align with fasting hours. This allows for adequate absorption while avoiding interference with the fast.
- **Hydration**: Proper hydration during non-fasting hours is essential, as dehydration can increase the risk of seizures. Encourage patients to drink plenty of fluids between Iftar and Suhoor.
- **Monitoring**: Patients should be closely monitored for signs of breakthrough seizures or side effects, particularly during the first few days of fasting when medication levels may fluctuate.

Anticonvulsant Medications and

Timing Adjustments

Carbamazepine

Carbamazepine is commonly used to treat partial and generalized seizures. Since it has a long half-life, dosing adjustments during Ramadan may be necessary to maintain consistent drug levels.

Drug Name	Timing Recommendation	Notes
Carbamazepine (IR)	After Iftar and before or with Suhoor	Redistribute doses to keep steady plasma levels. Larger dose at Iftar, smaller dose at Suhoor.
Carbamazepine (MR)	After Iftar and before or with Suhoor	Controlled-release formulation allows for once-daily dosing; take after Iftar.

Levetiracetam

Levetiracetam is another common anticonvulsant used for seizure control. It can be taken twice daily, and adjustments are made based on the patient's schedule during Ramadan.

Drug Name	Timing Recommendation	Notes
Levetiracetam	After Iftar and before or with Suhoor	Can be taken at the same time every day to avoid missed doses.
Levetiracetam (XR)	After Iftar and before or with Suhoor	Extended-release formulation is preferred for once-daily dosing.

Valproate

Valproate is commonly used for generalized and partial seizures.

It is typically taken twice a day, and dosing adjustments should be made to prevent hypoglycemia and maintain consistent blood levels.

Drug Name	Timing Recommendation	Notes
Valproate (IR)	After Iftar and before or with Suhoor	Ensure regular blood level monitoring to avoid toxicity.
Valproate (XR)	After Iftar and before or with Suhoor	Extended-release formulation is useful for once-daily dosing.

Additional Anticonvulsant Medications

Lamotrigine

Lamotrigine is used to treat partial seizures and generalized tonic-clonic seizures. It is generally well-tolerated and may require dose adjustments during fasting to prevent the risk of breakthrough seizures.

Drug Name	Timing Recommendation	Notes
Lamotrigine	After Iftar and before or with Suhoor	Ensure regular dosing schedule to maintain therapeutic levels.

Phenytoin

Phenytoin is an effective anticonvulsant for preventing generalized tonic-clonic seizures and partial seizures. Due to its narrow therapeutic range, dosing adjustments are crucial to avoid toxicity.

Drug Name	Timing Recommendation	Notes

| Phenytoin | After Iftar and before or with Suhoor | Monitor plasma levels regularly to avoid toxicity. |

General Advice for Epilepsy Medications During Ramadan

1. **Consistent Timing**: Ensure medications are taken consistently at the same times each day, ideally after Iftar and before or with Suhoor. This minimizes fluctuations in drug levels that could lead to breakthrough seizures.
2. **Adherence**: Patients must adhere strictly to their prescribed regimen. Missing doses can increase the risk of seizures, particularly during Ramadan when fasting can alter their regular routine.
3. **Hydration**: Encourage patients to hydrate adequately between Iftar and Suhoor to prevent dehydration, which can increase the risk of seizures.
4. **Seizure Monitoring**: Patients should be monitored for any signs of breakthrough seizures or other side effects. If seizures occur during Ramadan, medication adjustments or further consultation with the healthcare provider may be necessary.
5. **Avoiding Triggers**: Certain foods, stress, or lack of sleep can trigger seizures. Patients should be advised to avoid known triggers during fasting and to maintain a regular sleep schedule.

Special Considerations for Specific Patient Groups

Elderly Patients

- Elderly patients may have altered drug metabolism, making them more susceptible to side effects and toxicity. Dosing may need to be adjusted, and regular monitoring is essential.

- These patients are also at higher risk for dehydration and should be monitored closely during Ramadan.

Children

- Children with epilepsy may require adjusted doses and should be closely monitored for any changes in seizure frequency during fasting.
- Ensure that younger patients understand the importance of medication adherence and hydration.

Key Takeaways for Epilepsy Medications During Ramadan:

1. **Timing**: Anticonvulsants should be taken **after Iftar and before or with Suhoor** to ensure steady drug levels and minimize the risk of seizures.
2. **Hydration**: Encourage adequate hydration between Iftar and Suhoor to prevent dehydration, which can trigger seizures.
3. **Monitoring**: Patients should regularly monitor their seizure activity and report any breakthrough seizures or side effects.
4. **Adherence**: Consistency is key—missed doses can lead to increased seizure risk. Patients must adhere to their prescribed regimen without alteration

CHAPTER 7: HYPERLIPIDEMIA AND LIPID-LOWERING AGENTS

Hyperlipidemia, or high cholesterol, is a common condition treated with lipid-lowering medications such as statins, fibrates, and bile acid sequestrants. Managing lipid levels during Ramadan is crucial for preventing cardiovascular complications, especially for patients with a history of heart disease or diabetes. This chapter covers common lipid-lowering medications, with a focus on adjusting their timing and ensuring their effectiveness during fasting.

General Considerations for Lipid-Lowering Medications

- **Timing**: Lipid-lowering agents should be taken **after Iftar and before or with Suhoor** to align with fasting hours and ensure optimal absorption.
- **Hydration**: Some lipid-lowering medications, such as fibrates, can increase the risk of dehydration and should be taken with adequate fluids during non-fasting hours.
- **Consistency**: Patients should continue their medication regimen as prescribed, without skipping doses. For medications requiring adjustments, patients should consult their healthcare provider for proper guidance.

Statins

Statins are the most commonly prescribed medication for managing high cholesterol. They work by inhibiting the enzyme HMG-CoA reductase, which plays a key role in cholesterol production. Statins are typically well-tolerated, but their timing and dose adjustments may be necessary during Ramadan.

Drug Name	Timing Recommendation	Notes
Atorvastatin (Long-acting)	After Iftar and before or with Suhoor	Best taken in the evening, as this is when cholesterol production peaks.
Rosuvastatin (Long-acting)	After Iftar and before or with Suhoor	Consistent timing helps to maintain drug efficacy.
Simvastatin (Short-acting)	After Iftar and before or with Suhoor	Can be taken in the evening, but avoid taking with grapefruit juice.
Pravastatin (Short-acting)	After Iftar and before or with Suhoor	Less interaction with food and other medications.

General Advice for Statins:

- **Timing**: Statins are generally best taken **after Iftar and before or with Suhoor**, especially short-acting versions. Long-acting statins can be taken after Iftar for consistent effects.
- **Avoid Grapefruit**: Grapefruit juice can interfere with statin metabolism, particularly with medications like simvastatin, and should be avoided.
- **Side Effects**: Monitor for muscle pain or weakness, which can be a side effect of statins, particularly when used in combination with other medications that affect muscle function.

Fibrates

Fibrates are often prescribed to reduce triglyceride levels and increase HDL (good cholesterol). These medications work by activating peroxisome proliferator-activated receptors (PPARs) to break down lipids in the bloodstream. Fibrates may need to be adjusted for timing and hydration during Ramadan.

Drug Name	Timing Recommendation	Notes
Fenofibrate	After Iftar and before or with Suhoor	Take with food to improve absorption and reduce stomach upset.
Gemfibrozil	After Iftar and before or with Suhoor	Ensure adequate hydration as dehydration can increase the risk of side effects.

General Advice for Fibrates:
- **Hydration**: These medications can cause dehydration, so it is essential to drink plenty of fluids during non-fasting hours.
- **Food Intake**: Fibrates should be taken with food (after Iftar) to enhance absorption and reduce gastrointestinal side effects like nausea and stomach discomfort.

Bile Acid Sequestrants

Bile acid sequestrants like cholestyramine work by binding to bile acids in the intestines, preventing their reabsorption. This process helps to lower LDL (bad cholesterol) levels. These medications should be taken with meals for optimal effect.

Drug Name	Timing Recommendation	Notes
Cholestyramine	After Iftar and before or	Take with food to avoid

	with Suhoor	gastrointestinal discomfort.
Colesevelam	After Iftar and before or with Suhoor	Can be taken with meals for improved efficacy and reduced gastrointestinal side effects.

General Advice for Bile Acid Sequestrants:

- **Timing**: Take these medications **after Iftar and before or with Suhoor** to ensure proper absorption, especially when taken with food.
- **Side Effects**: Patients may experience bloating or constipation, so adequate hydration and fiber intake are recommended during Ramadan.

Other Lipid-Lowering Medications

Ezetimibe

Ezetimibe works by inhibiting cholesterol absorption in the intestines. It is often prescribed in combination with statins for added effect.

Drug Name	Timing Recommendation	Notes
Ezetimibe	After Iftar and before or with Suhoor	Can be taken with or without food; adjust timing based on patient preference.

PCSK9 Inhibitors

PCSK9 inhibitors are a newer class of injectable medications used to lower LDL cholesterol levels. These medications are typically prescribed for patients with high cardiovascular risk and those who cannot tolerate statins.

Drug Name	Timing Recommendation	Notes
Alirocumab	After Iftar and before or with Suhoor	Administer according to prescribed schedule; typically given every two weeks.
Evolocumab	After Iftar and before or with Suhoor	Similar to alirocumab, take during non-fasting hours.

Managing Lipid-Lowering Medications During Ramadan

1. **Consistency**: Patients should take their medications consistently at the same time each day, ideally **after Iftar and before or with Suhoor**.
2. **Hydration**: Ensure that patients drink plenty of water during non-fasting hours, especially when taking fibrates, which can increase the risk of dehydration.
3. **Dietary Considerations**: Encourage a heart-healthy diet with plenty of vegetables, lean proteins, and whole grains during non-fasting hours to support the effectiveness of lipid-lowering medications.
4. **Monitoring**: Regular monitoring of cholesterol levels and potential side effects, such as muscle pain or gastrointestinal discomfort, is important during Ramadan.

Key Takeaways for Lipid-Lowering Medications During Ramadan:

1. **Timing**: Most lipid-lowering medications, including statins, fibrates, and bile acid sequestrants, should be

taken **after Iftar and before or with Suhoor** to optimize their effectiveness while minimizing side effects.
2. **Hydration**: Ensure that patients remain well-hydrated during the non-fasting hours to prevent dehydration-related side effects, especially with fibrates.
3. **Adherence**: Patients should continue taking their lipid-lowering medications as prescribed, and consult with their healthcare provider if they experience any adverse effects or need adjustments during Ramadan.
4. **Dietary Adjustments**: Advise patients to avoid high-fat, high-cholesterol foods during Iftar and Suhoor to enhance the effectiveness of lipid-lowering therapies.

CHAPTER 8: ANTICOAGULANTS

Anticoagulants are used to prevent blood clots in patients with conditions such as atrial fibrillation, deep vein thrombosis (DVT), and pulmonary embolism (PE). While fasting during Ramadan, adjustments to anticoagulant regimens may be necessary to ensure both the effectiveness of the medication and the safety of the patient. This chapter outlines the recommended adjustments for commonly used anticoagulants, with a focus on timing, monitoring, and special considerations during Ramadan.

General Considerations for Anticoagulants During Ramadan

- **Timing**: Anticoagulants should be taken **after Iftar and before or with Suhoor** to ensure that they are absorbed properly and to minimize the risk of bleeding during fasting hours.
- **Hydration**: Adequate hydration is essential when using anticoagulants, as dehydration can lead to concentration changes in the blood, increasing the risk of clotting or bleeding.
- **Monitoring**: Regular monitoring of the patient's INR (for warfarin) or other clotting markers is crucial to ensure therapeutic levels are maintained during fasting.

Warfarin

Warfarin is a commonly prescribed oral anticoagulant that works by inhibiting vitamin K-dependent clotting factors. Because of its narrow therapeutic index, regular monitoring of INR is essential to ensure that the patient remains within the therapeutic range.

Drug Name	Timing Recommendation	Notes
Warfarin	After Iftar and before or with Suhoor	Ensure INR is monitored regularly, as fasting and changes in diet can affect INR levels.
Warfarin (adjusted dose)	After Iftar and before or with Suhoor	Adjust doses based on INR results, ensuring therapeutic anticoagulation during fasting.

General Advice for Warfarin:

- **Dietary Considerations**: Patients should be advised to maintain a consistent diet with regard to vitamin K-rich foods (e.g., leafy greens) to avoid fluctuations in INR levels.
- **INR Monitoring**: Regular INR testing should be done, particularly during the first few days of Ramadan, to adjust the dose as needed.
- **Hydration**: Ensure that patients are properly hydrated to prevent fluctuations in INR caused by dehydration.

Direct Oral Anticoagulants (DOACs)

Direct oral anticoagulants (DOACs), such as apixaban, rivaroxaban, and dabigatran, are becoming increasingly popular due to their more predictable pharmacokinetics and lack of need for routine monitoring (compared to warfarin). However, dosing adjustments and timing considerations are still necessary during Ramadan.

Apixaban (Eliquis)

Apixaban is commonly prescribed for stroke prevention in atrial fibrillation and for treating DVT and PE. It is a direct factor Xa inhibitor.

Drug Name	Timing Recommendation	Notes
Apixaban	After Iftar and before or with Suhoor	Can be taken once or twice daily depending on the prescribed regimen.

Rivaroxaban (Xarelto)

Rivaroxaban is also a factor Xa inhibitor and is typically prescribed for the prevention and treatment of DVT, PE, and stroke prevention in atrial fibrillation.

Drug Name	Timing Recommendation	Notes
Rivaroxaban	After Iftar and before or with Suhoor	Take with food to enhance absorption. For once-daily dosing, ensure consistent timing.

Dabigatran (Pradaxa)

Dabigatran is a direct thrombin inhibitor used to reduce the risk of stroke in atrial fibrillation and to treat DVT and PE.

Drug Name	Timing Recommendation	Notes
Dabigatran	After Iftar and before or with Suhoor	Take with food to minimize gastrointestinal irritation.

General Advice for DOACs:

- **Timing**: DOACs should be taken **after Iftar and before or with Suhoor** to optimize absorption and effectiveness.
- **Food Interaction**: Most DOACs should be taken with food to improve absorption. Ensure patients are advised to take these medications during the non-fasting hours, with meals, to maximize their effect.

- **Hydration**: Encourage adequate hydration to avoid dehydration, which can affect drug concentrations and increase the risk of clotting or bleeding.

Low Molecular Weight Heparin (LMWH)

LMWH, such as enoxaparin, is often used for the prevention of DVT in hospitalized patients or for managing acute conditions like PE. It is typically administered by subcutaneous injection.

Drug Name	Timing Recommendation	Notes
Enoxaparin	After Iftar and before or with Suhoor	Administered by subcutaneous injection; follow prescribed schedule carefully.

General Advice for LMWH:

- **Injection Timing**: For patients on LMWH, it is important to maintain the prescribed injection schedule. Injections are typically given once or twice a day and should be administered **after Iftar and before or with Suhoor** to avoid any disruption to the fasting schedule.
- **Monitoring**: Patients on LMWH should have regular monitoring of their anti-Xa levels to ensure therapeutic dosing.
- **Hydration**: Adequate hydration is essential when using injectable anticoagulants to prevent dehydration, which can impact the medication's effectiveness.

Antiplatelet Medications

Antiplatelet medications, such as aspirin and clopidogrel, are commonly prescribed for patients at risk of cardiovascular events, such as stroke or heart attack. These medications should be taken with food to minimize gastrointestinal irritation.

Drug Name	Timing Recommendation	Notes
Aspirin	After Iftar and before or with Suhoor	Take with food to minimize stomach irritation.
Clopidogrel	After Iftar and before or with Suhoor	Ensure that it is taken consistently to maintain antiplatelet effects.

General Advice for Antiplatelets:

- **Timing**: Antiplatelet medications should be taken **after Iftar and before or with Suhoor** to ensure optimal absorption and to avoid gastric irritation.
- **Food**: These medications should be taken with food, especially aspirin, to reduce the risk of gastrointestinal bleeding.

Key Takeaways for Anticoagulants During Ramadan:

1. **Timing**: Most anticoagulants, including warfarin, DOACs, and LMWH, should be taken **after Iftar and before or with Suhoor** to ensure optimal absorption and therapeutic efficacy.
2. **Hydration**: Adequate hydration is essential to prevent dehydration-related complications, especially for patients on warfarin and DOACs.
3. **Monitoring**: Regular monitoring of INR (for warfarin) or anti-Xa levels (for LMWH) is crucial during Ramadan to ensure that patients remain within therapeutic ranges.
4. **Adherence**: Patients should adhere strictly to the prescribed dosing regimen to minimize the risk of bleeding or clotting. Missing doses or adjusting doses without consulting a healthcare provider can lead to serious complications.

CHAPTER 9: ASTHMA MANAGEMENT DURING RAMADAN

Asthma is a chronic respiratory condition characterized by inflammation and narrowing of the airways, leading to symptoms like wheezing, shortness of breath, and coughing. Managing asthma during Ramadan can be challenging, particularly when it comes to medication timing and potential asthma triggers. This chapter provides recommendations on adjusting asthma medications to ensure optimal symptom control during fasting Inhalers are generally considered to be acceptable during fasting, but there are differing opinions among Muslim scholars:Some scholars say that using an inhaler is not the same as eating or drinking, and is therefore permitted during fasting.Some scholars say that inhalers provide small amounts of liquid medicine to the lungs, so they break the fast.

General Considerations for Asthma Medications During Ramadan

- **Timing**: Asthma medications should be taken **after Iftar and before or with Suhoor**, particularly inhalers and oral medications, to avoid disrupting the fast and ensure effective symptom management.
- **Hydration**: Staying well-hydrated during non-fasting hours is crucial to help prevent airway dryness and reduce the risk of asthma attacks.

- **Peak Flow Monitoring**: Patients should use a peak flow meter to monitor their lung function and adjust medications as necessary.

Inhalers: Short-acting and Long-acting

Inhalers are the cornerstone of asthma management, with two main categories: short-acting bronchodilators for quick relief and long-acting bronchodilators for maintenance treatment. The timing and use of inhalers during fasting need to be adjusted for both effectiveness and convenience.

Short-Acting Beta-Agonists (SABAs)

Short-acting beta-agonists, such as salbutamol (albuterol), are used for quick relief of asthma symptoms, providing rapid bronchodilation during an asthma attack or wheezing.

Drug Name	Timing Recommendation	Notes
Salbutamol (Albuterol)	As needed after Iftar or before Suhoor	Use as a rescue inhaler when experiencing symptoms.
Terbutaline	As needed after Iftar or before Suhoor	Effective for acute symptom relief. Avoid overuse.

Long-Acting Beta-Agonists (LABAs)

LABAs are used for maintaining long-term asthma control by helping to relax the muscles around the airways and prevent symptoms. These medications are usually taken once or twice a day.

Drug Name	Timing Recommendation	Notes
Salmeterol	After Iftar and before or with Suhoor	Typically used with inhaled corticosteroids for better control.
Formoterol	After Iftar and before or	Combine with

	with Suhoor	corticosteroids for effective asthma control.

Inhaled Corticosteroids (ICS)

Inhaled corticosteroids are the most effective long-term treatment for asthma, helping to reduce inflammation in the airways and prevent asthma attacks. These should be taken consistently as prescribed, with doses adjusted to ensure continuous control.

Drug Name	Timing Recommendation	Notes
Fluticasone	After Iftar and before or with Suhoor	Take with a spacer if needed to improve inhalation technique.
Budesonide	After Iftar and before or with Suhoor	Can be combined with LABAs for optimal control.
Beclometasone	After Iftar and before or with Suhoor	Ensure proper inhalation technique to reduce oral side effects.

Combination Inhalers (ICS + LABA)

Combination inhalers, which combine an inhaled corticosteroid with a long-acting beta-agonist, offer the benefit of improved asthma control with a single inhaler. These medications are typically used twice daily.

Drug Name	Timing Recommendation	Notes
Seretide (Fluticasone + Salmeterol)	After Iftar and before or with Suhoor	Provides long-acting relief for both inflammation and bronchoconstriction.
Symbicort (Budesonide + Formoterol)	After Iftar and before or with Suhoor	Fast-acting formoterol provides relief from acute

		symptoms.

Oral Medications for Asthma

For patients with more severe asthma, oral medications such as leukotriene receptor antagonists and corticosteroids may be used as additional therapies. Adjusting the timing of these medications ensures continuous asthma control without disrupting the fasting routine.

Leukotriene Receptor Antagonists (LTRAs)

Leukotrienes are chemicals in the body that cause inflammation in the airways, leading to asthma symptoms. LTRAs work by blocking the action of these chemicals.

Drug Name	Timing Recommendation	Notes
Montelukast	After Iftar and before or with Suhoor	Take once daily; helps to prevent nighttime asthma symptoms.

Oral Corticosteroids

Oral corticosteroids are typically used for short-term control during asthma exacerbations or flare-ups. These medications help to reduce airway inflammation.

Drug Name	Timing Recommendation	Notes
Prednisolone	After Iftar and before or with Suhoor	Typically used for short periods, especially during flare-ups.
Methylprednisolone	After Iftar and before or with Suhoor	Used for more severe asthma exacerbations.

Managing Asthma Exacerbations During Ramadan

Asthma exacerbations can occur due to several factors, including exposure to allergens, dehydration, or changes in routine. During Ramadan, managing asthma exacerbations requires rapid and effective treatment, as well as preventing triggers during fasting hours.

1. **Recognizing Symptoms**: Patients should be advised to recognize early signs of asthma exacerbation, such as increased wheezing, shortness of breath, or frequent coughing. Immediate use of a short-acting beta-agonist (e.g., salbutamol) is essential.
2. **Action Plan**: Ensure patients have a written asthma action plan that includes instructions on medication use during exacerbations, as well as when to seek emergency medical help.
3. **Triggers**: Avoid common asthma triggers such as strong perfumes, smoke, and foods that may cause acid reflux or allergens during fasting hours.

Special Considerations for Asthma Medications During Ramadan

Elderly Patients

- Elderly patients may require adjustments to the dosing of inhaled corticosteroids and bronchodilators. They may also have a higher risk of side effects such as oral thrush or hoarseness from inhaled steroids.
- Ensure proper inhalation technique, and consider the use of a spacer with inhalers to maximize delivery of the medication.

Children

- For pediatric asthma patients, it is essential to ensure

that they are properly trained in inhaler techniques and understand the importance of medication adherence.
- Children may need additional support to adjust their medication regimen during Ramadan, particularly if they are fasting.

Key Takeaways for Asthma Management During Ramadan:

1. **Timing**: Asthma medications, including inhalers (SABAs, LABAs, ICS), and oral medications (LTRAs, corticosteroids) should be taken **after Iftar and before or with Suhoor** to avoid disrupting the fast and maintain asthma control.
2. **Hydration**: Proper hydration is essential during non-fasting hours to keep airways moist and reduce the risk of asthma attacks.
3. **Monitoring**: Regular monitoring of asthma symptoms and peak flow measurements is important to ensure asthma control during fasting.
4. **Adherence**: Consistent adherence to the prescribed medication regimen is critical to managing asthma effectively during Ramadan.

CHAPTER 10: THYROID CONDITIONS AND HORMONAL THERAPIES

Thyroid conditions, including hypothyroidism and hyperthyroidism, are common and require lifelong medication. Fasting during Ramadan may affect medication timing and absorption, making it important to adjust thyroid medications to ensure optimal hormonal balance. This chapter provides guidance on managing thyroid conditions during Ramadan, focusing on timing adjustments for thyroid hormone replacement therapy (THRT) and medications for hyperthyroidism.

General Considerations for Thyroid Medications During Ramadan

- **Timing**: Thyroid medications, particularly thyroid hormone replacement (e.g., levothyroxine), should be taken **before Suhoor** on an empty stomach for optimal absorption. Medications for hyperthyroidism, such as carbimazole, should be taken **after Iftar and before or with Suhoor** to maintain steady drug levels.
- **Hydration**: Proper hydration is essential for all thyroid medications, especially for patients on thyroid hormone replacement, as dehydration can affect drug metabolism.

- **Consistency**: Consistency in medication timing is important, especially for thyroid hormone replacement. Patients should avoid altering the timing of doses without consulting their healthcare provider.

Hypothyroidism and Thyroid Hormone Replacement

Hypothyroidism occurs when the thyroid gland produces insufficient thyroid hormones, leading to symptoms such as fatigue, weight gain, and cold intolerance. The standard treatment is thyroid hormone replacement therapy (THRT), typically with levothyroxine.

Levothyroxine

Levothyroxine is a synthetic form of the thyroid hormone thyroxine (T4), which helps normalize thyroid hormone levels and maintain proper metabolic function.

Drug Name	Timing Recommendation	Notes
Levothyroxine	Before Suhoor, on an empty stomach	Take at least 30–60 minutes before Suhoor for optimal absorption. Avoid food, coffee, and calcium supplements for 30 minutes after taking the medication.
Levothyroxine (liquid form)	Before Suhoor, on an empty stomach	Same timing as tablet form, ensuring there are no food or drink interactions.

General Advice for Hypothyroidism Medications:

- **Food Interaction**: Levothyroxine is best absorbed on an empty stomach. Patients should take their medication **before Suhoor** and avoid eating or drinking anything except

water for at least 30 minutes after the dose.
- **Hydration**: Encourage patients to drink water after taking their thyroid medication to aid absorption.
- **Consistency**: Patients should take their thyroid medication at the same time every day during Ramadan to maintain consistent thyroid hormone levels.

Hyperthyroidism and Antithyroid Medications

Hyperthyroidism occurs when the thyroid produces excessive amounts of thyroid hormones, leading to symptoms such as rapid heart rate, weight loss, and nervousness. The main treatments for hyperthyroidism are antithyroid medications such as carbimazole or propylthiouracil (PTU), which reduce thyroid hormone production.

Carbimazole

Carbimazole is the most commonly used medication for hyperthyroidism. It works by inhibiting the synthesis of thyroid hormones in the thyroid gland.

Drug Name	Timing Recommendation	Notes
Carbimazole	After Iftar and before or with Suhoor	Take with food to reduce gastrointestinal side effects.

Propylthiouracil (PTU)

Propylthiouracil (PTU) is another antithyroid medication used to treat hyperthyroidism. It works by inhibiting the conversion of T4 to T3, reducing the amount of active thyroid hormone in the body.

Drug Name	Timing Recommendation	Notes
Propylthiouracil (PTU)	After Iftar and before or with Suhoor	Take with food to minimize stomach irritation.

General Advice for Hyperthyroidism Medications:

- **Timing**: Antithyroid medications such as carbimazole and PTU should be taken **after Iftar and before or with Suhoor** to ensure effective drug absorption while aligning with fasting hours.
- **Food**: These medications should be taken with food to reduce gastrointestinal discomfort and ensure better absorption.
- **Regular Monitoring**: Regular blood tests are essential for patients on antithyroid medications to monitor thyroid hormone levels and prevent complications such as hypothyroidism.

Managing Thyroid Conditions During Ramadan

1. **Consistency**: It is crucial that patients with thyroid conditions take their medications consistently and at the same times every day during Ramadan. Missed doses or inconsistent timing can lead to fluctuations in thyroid hormone levels.
2. **Hydration**: Proper hydration is important for thyroid hormone metabolism. Patients should drink plenty of water during non-fasting hours to prevent dehydration, which can affect the absorption of thyroid medication.
3. **Monitoring**: Regular monitoring of thyroid function is recommended to ensure that patients remain euthyroid (normal thyroid function) during Ramadan, particularly if any dose adjustments are made.

Special Considerations for Thyroid Medications During Ramadan

Elderly Patients

- Elderly patients may experience slower metabolism and may require dose adjustments for both thyroid hormone replacement and antithyroid medications. Careful

monitoring is essential to avoid under- or over-treatment.
- Older patients may also be at higher risk for dehydration, which can affect thyroid hormone levels. Ensure they remain well-hydrated.

Pregnancy and Breastfeeding
- Pregnant women or those breastfeeding who have thyroid conditions should consult their healthcare provider before making any changes to their thyroid medication regimen during Ramadan. Pregnancy can affect thyroid function, and adjustments may be necessary to maintain proper thyroid hormone levels.

Key Takeaways for Thyroid Medications During Ramadan:

1. **Timing**: Thyroid medications should be taken **before Suhoor** (on an empty stomach) for hypothyroidism and **after Iftar and before or with Suhoor** for hyperthyroidism treatments.
2. **Hydration**: Adequate hydration between Iftar and Suhoor is essential for optimal thyroid medication absorption and metabolism.
3. **Consistency**: Consistency in medication timing is crucial for managing thyroid conditions. Patients should stick to their prescribed regimen without making adjustments without consulting their healthcare provider.
4. **Monitoring**: Regular monitoring of thyroid function, particularly for patients on antithyroid medications, is important during Ramadan to ensure balanced thyroid hormone levels and avoid complications.

Hormone Replacement Therapy (HRT) Considerations During Ramadan

Medication Type	Examples	Timing Considerations	Side Effects	Special Considerations
Estrogen Therapy	Estradiol, Conjugated	Take **after Iftar** (with	Nausea, bloating,	Ensure hydration,

	Estrogens (Premarin)	food) for optimal absorption	headaches, weight gain	particularly for those with a history of fluid retention or cardiovascular disease. May cause bloating, especially when fasting.
Progesterone Therapy	Medroxyprogesterone acetate, Norethindrone	Take **after Iftar** to minimize nausea	Mood swings, dizziness, headaches	Progesterone can cause mood swings or irritability. Timing it post-Iftar helps alleviate gastrointestinal discomfort and fatigue.
Combined HRT	Estradiol + Norethindrone (e.g., Activella)	Take **after Iftar** or **before Suhoor**	Nausea, bloating, irritability, weight gain	For combined HRT, ensure that it is taken with food to avoid GI upset. Adjust for any side effects affecting fasting, such as mood swings.
Transdermal Estrogen	Estradiol patches, gels	Apply **after Iftar** (typically done once or twice a week)	Skin irritation, headaches	Transdermal forms bypass the digestive system, making them less likely to cause GI distress. Hydration is still important, as dehydration can impact skin absorption.
Bioidentical HRT	Micronized progesterone, Estradiol cream	Apply **after Iftar**, similar to transdermal options	Sleep disturbances, mood swings	Bioidentical HRT is often seen as a more natural alternative but should still be managed with attention to hydration and side effects like mood changes during Ramadan.
Testosterone Therapy (for women)	Testosterone cypionate, Testosterone patches	Apply **after Iftar** or **before Suhoor**	Acne, hair growth, mood swings	Consider the risk of side effects such as acne or excessive hair growth. Patients should consult their doctor to ensure the correct timing relative to fasting hours.

Key Notes for Managing HRT During Ramadan:

- **Medication Timing**: The general recommendation is to take oral HRT **after Iftar**, with food, to reduce the likelihood of nausea or gastrointestinal upset. If the medication is once-daily, it should ideally be taken in the evening after Iftar to align with the patient's fasting schedule. For transdermal or patch forms, the medication may be applied at any time of day, but after Iftar is preferable to ensure comfort.
- **Hydration**: Maintaining hydration during non-fasting hours is critical, as HRT can sometimes cause fluid retention. Encourage patients to drink plenty of water between Iftar and Suhoor.
- **Side Effect Management**: If patients experience mood swings, bloating, or irritability while fasting, advise them to adjust the medication timing or consult their healthcare provider for possible adjustments. The fasting period may

exacerbate fatigue or mood disturbances, particularly for patients on combined or progesterone-only therapy.
- **Monitoring**: Women on HRT should have regular follow-ups with their healthcare provider to ensure that the treatment plan remains effective, especially during Ramadan when fasting can affect medication absorption and metabolism.

CHAPTER 11: ANTIVIRALS AND RETROVIRALS

Antiviral and retroviral medications are critical for treating infections caused by viruses, such as influenza, HIV, and hepatitis. Fasting during Ramadan presents unique challenges when managing these medications, as it requires adjustments to timing and dosage to maintain their effectiveness while respecting the fasting routine. This chapter outlines strategies for managing antiviral and retroviral medications during Ramadan, focusing on their timing, interactions, and special considerations.

General Considerations for Antivirals and Retrovirals During Ramadan

- **Timing**: Most antiviral and retroviral medications should be taken **after Iftar and before or with Suhoor** to ensure proper absorption and to minimize the risk of side effects during fasting hours.
- **Hydration**: Staying well-hydrated between Iftar and Suhoor is essential, particularly for medications that may cause dehydration or gastrointestinal side effects.
- **Adherence**: Adherence to the prescribed regimen is crucial to avoid resistance, especially for HIV and hepatitis treatments. Patients should not skip doses during Ramadan.

Antivirals for Acute Infections

Antivirals are used to treat acute viral infections such as influenza, herpes simplex virus (HSV), and hepatitis C. Proper timing and adherence are essential to ensuring effectiveness.

Oseltamivir (Tamiflu)

Oseltamivir is commonly prescribed for the treatment and prevention of influenza. It is most effective when started early in the course of infection.

Drug Name	Timing Recommendation	Notes
Oseltamivir	After Iftar and before or with Suhoor	Take for five days if prescribed for influenza treatment. It can be taken with or without food.

Acyclovir

Acyclovir is commonly used to treat herpes simplex virus (HSV) infections, including cold sores and genital herpes.

Drug Name	Timing Recommendation	Notes
Acyclovir	After Iftar and before or with Suhoor	Ensure complete course is followed to reduce the risk of recurrence.

General Advice for Antivirals:

- **Timing**: For most antivirals, taking the medication **after Iftar and before or with Suhoor** helps maintain proper blood concentrations and prevents interference with fasting hours.
- Side Effects: Some antivirals, such as oseltamivir, can cause gastrointestinal upset. Take these medications with food to minimize side effects.
- **Hydration**: Hydration is important, especially when

using antivirals for systemic infections, as some can lead to dehydration.

Retrovirals for Chronic Infections (HIV, Hepatitis)

Retroviral medications are essential for the management of chronic viral infections like HIV and hepatitis B/C. These medications require strict adherence to avoid viral resistance and to ensure optimal therapeutic effect. Timing and food interactions are key factors in managing these medications during Ramadan.

Tenofovir (HIV, Hepatitis B)

Tenofovir is used to treat HIV and chronic hepatitis B. It is a nucleotide reverse transcriptase inhibitor (NRTI) that helps prevent the replication of the virus.

Drug Name	Timing Recommendation	Notes
Tenofovir	After Iftar and before or with Suhoor	Can be taken with or without food. Patients should take the full prescribed dose.

Dolutegravir (HIV)

Dolutegravir is an integrase strand transfer inhibitor (INSTI) used in combination therapy for HIV.

Drug Name	Timing Recommendation	Notes

| Dolutegravir | After Iftar and before or with Suhoor | Can be taken with or without food, once daily. |

Ritonavir (HIV)

Ritonavir is a protease inhibitor used in the treatment of HIV, often as part of a combination regimen.

Drug Name	Timing Recommendation	Notes
Ritonavir	After Iftar and before or with Suhoor	Take with food to avoid gastrointestinal upset.

General Advice for Retroviral Medications:

- **Timing**: Retrovirals should be taken **after Iftar and before or with Suhoor** to avoid disrupting the fasting hours and to optimize drug absorption.
- **Consistency**: Adherence to the prescribed regimen is critical to avoid viral resistance and maintain therapeutic drug levels. Missing doses can significantly reduce the effectiveness of retroviral therapy.
- **Hydration**: Adequate hydration is important, particularly for medications like tenofovir, which can affect kidney function. Encourage patients to drink plenty of fluids during non-fasting hours.

Special Considerations for Antivirals and Retrovirals During Ramadan

Elderly Patients

- Elderly patients may have slower drug metabolism and altered renal function, making it important to adjust dosing regimens for antiviral and retroviral medications accordingly. Careful monitoring of kidney and liver function

is recommended.
- These patients are also at higher risk of dehydration and should be monitored closely for any signs of electrolyte imbalances or adverse drug reactions.

Pregnancy and Breastfeeding
- Pregnant or breastfeeding women who are on antiviral or retroviral therapy should consult their healthcare provider before Ramadan to ensure that their medications are appropriate and safe during fasting.
- For HIV-positive pregnant women, maintaining a stable viral load is essential to avoid mother-to-child transmission, and they should not alter their medication schedule during Ramadan.

HIV Patients with Co-morbidities
- HIV patients who are also managing other conditions (such as tuberculosis or hepatitis) should be closely monitored for drug interactions, particularly when using multiple medications. Adjustments may be needed based on the patient's overall health and medication regimen.

Key Takeaways for Antivirals and Retrovirals During Ramadan:

1. **Timing**: Antiviral and retroviral medications should be taken **after Iftar and before or with Suhoor** to align with fasting hours and optimize absorption.
2. **Hydration**: Encourage proper hydration between Iftar and Suhoor, as dehydration can impact the efficacy of antiviral and retroviral treatments.
3. **Adherence**: Patients should adhere strictly to their prescribed medication schedule to avoid treatment failure and viral resistance.
4. **Monitoring**: Regular monitoring of renal and liver function is recommended, particularly for long-term

users of medications like tenofovir or ritonavir, to prevent complications.

CHAPTER 12: CANCER MEDICATIONS AND MANAGEMENT

Cancer treatment often involves a combination of therapies aimed at slowing or halting the progression of cancer cells. These treatments include surgery, radiation, and various forms of chemotherapy, immunotherapy, targeted therapy, and hormone therapy. As cancer medications can be quite complex and vary depending on the type of cancer and its stage, managing these treatments during Ramadan requires careful consideration to ensure patient safety, particularly regarding fasting.

1. Chemotherapy

Chemotherapy is a treatment that uses powerful drugs to kill cancer cells or stop their growth. Chemotherapy can be administered orally, intravenously, or through other routes. The main aim of chemotherapy is to target and destroy rapidly dividing cancer cells.

Types of Chemotherapy Drugs

- **Alkylating Agents**: These drugs work by interfering with DNA replication in cancer cells. Common examples include cyclophosphamide, ifosfamide, and chlorambucil.
- **Antimetabolites**: These drugs mimic the building blocks of DNA and RNA, blocking cancer cells from reproducing. Examples include methotrexate, 5-fluorouracil (5-FU), and cytarabine.

- **Anthracyclines**: Used for several types of cancer, these drugs include doxorubicin and daunorubicin, which interfere with DNA replication.
- **Taxanes**: These drugs prevent cancer cells from dividing by interfering with microtubules, essential for cell division. Common drugs include paclitaxel and docetaxel.

Considerations During Ramadan

- **Timing of Doses**: Chemotherapy can cause severe nausea and fatigue. If chemotherapy is given intravenously or as a pill, the timing of doses should ideally be adjusted to fall **after Iftar and before Suhoor**, to minimize discomfort and dehydration.
- **Hydration**: Some chemotherapy drugs, particularly those that are intravenous, can cause dehydration, so it's important to monitor fluid intake during non-fasting hours.
- **Side Effects Management**: Chemotherapy often has side effects like nausea, vomiting, and fatigue. These side effects may be intensified when fasting. Patients should be educated on how to manage side effects and when to seek medical help.

2. Immunotherapy

Immunotherapy works by stimulating or enhancing the body's immune system to recognize and destroy cancer cells. These treatments can include monoclonal antibodies, checkpoint inhibitors, and cytokine therapy.

Types of Immunotherapy

- **Checkpoint Inhibitors**: These drugs block checkpoints (like PD-1 and PD-L1) that prevent immune cells from attacking cancer cells. Drugs like pembrolizumab and nivolumab are common examples.
- **Monoclonal Antibodies**: These lab-made molecules mimic the body's immune system and are designed to target

specific cancer antigens. Examples include rituximab and trastuzumab.
- **Cytokine Therapy**: Interleukins and interferons boost immune activity. These are less commonly used but can still be part of a treatment regimen.

Considerations During Ramadan

- **Timing and Administration**: Immunotherapy drugs can sometimes be administered intravenously in clinical settings. If the patient is undergoing outpatient therapy, the timing can be adjusted to align with **after Iftar**.
- **Fatigue**: Immunotherapy can cause fatigue, especially during the early weeks of treatment. Patients may feel weak during fasting hours, so it's essential to manage expectations and adjust doses if necessary.
- **Side Effects**: Patients undergoing immunotherapy may experience flu-like symptoms, fever, and rash. These should be addressed promptly, and medication schedules should be flexible, especially if side effects interfere with fasting.

3. Targeted Therapy

Targeted therapy uses drugs that specifically target cancer cell proteins or genes, and they work differently from standard chemotherapy. They tend to be more precise, affecting cancer cells without harming normal, healthy cells.

Types of Targeted Therapy

- **Tyrosine Kinase Inhibitors (TKIs)**: These drugs block enzymes that allow cancer cells to grow. Examples include imatinib (used for chronic myelogenous leukemia) and erlotinib (used for non-small cell lung cancer).
- **Monoclonal Antibodies**: Similar to those used in immunotherapy, monoclonal antibodies like rituximab can be used as part of targeted therapy.
- **Angiogenesis Inhibitors**: These drugs prevent the

formation of new blood vessels (angiogenesis) that tumors need to grow. Bevacizumab is one such example.

Considerations During Ramadan

- **Administration Schedule**: Many of these therapies can be taken orally, so adjusting the schedule to **after Iftar** is often possible. Intravenous therapies may require appointments, which should be scheduled outside of fasting hours.
- **Managing Side Effects**: Targeted therapies may cause side effects like skin rash, diarrhea, or liver issues. Patients should be informed about managing these side effects, especially when fasting may complicate hydration or medication timing.
- **Frequent Monitoring**: Some of these therapies require frequent blood tests to monitor liver and kidney function. This may need to be scheduled during non-fasting hours to ensure patient comfort.

4. Hormone Therapy

Hormone therapy is often used in cancers that are sensitive to hormones, such as breast, prostate, and ovarian cancers. These treatments work by blocking the body's ability to produce certain hormones or by interfering with the hormone-receptor interaction.

Types of Hormone Therapy

- **Aromatase Inhibitors**: Used primarily for breast cancer, these drugs lower estrogen levels, which can promote tumor growth. Examples include letrozole and anastrozole.
- **Selective Estrogen Receptor Modulators (SERMs)**: Tamoxifen is a commonly prescribed SERM that blocks estrogen receptors in breast cancer cells.
- **Luteinizing Hormone-Releasing Hormone (LHRH) Agonists**: Used for prostate cancer, these drugs decrease testosterone production. Examples include leuprolide.

Considerations During Ramadan

- **Timing**: Many hormone therapies are taken orally. If the patient is prescribed daily medications like tamoxifen or letrozole, these should be adjusted to **after Iftar** to ensure they are taken with food to reduce gastric irritation.
- **Side Effects**: Hormone therapy can cause side effects such as hot flashes, fatigue, and mood swings, which may be intensified during fasting. Managing these side effects with proper guidance is important.
- **Hydration**: Hormone therapy can lead to changes in hydration levels. Ensuring the patient remains hydrated during non-fasting hours is essential.

5. Palliative Care and Pain Management

For patients with advanced cancer, palliative care plays an important role in providing comfort and improving the quality of life. Pain management is a central component of palliative care.

Types of Pain Relief

- **Opioids**: Medications like morphine, oxycodone, and fentanyl are commonly used to control severe cancer pain.
- **Non-Opioid Analgesics**: Drugs like acetaminophen and NSAIDs (ibuprofen) are used for mild to moderate pain.

Considerations During Ramadan

- **Opioid Timing**: Opioid medications, which are typically taken on a regular schedule, can be adjusted to **after Iftar** for the best effect. However, some long-acting formulations can be given **before Suhoor** to provide relief throughout the day.
- **Managing Side Effects**: Pain medications can cause side effects such as constipation, drowsiness, or nausea, which may be compounded by fasting. Patients should be advised on how to manage these side effects, including the use of laxatives or anti-nausea medications.

Cancer medications are diverse, ranging from chemotherapy and immunotherapy to targeted therapies and hormone treatments. Managing these treatments during Ramadan requires careful planning, particularly in adjusting the timing of doses to align with fasting hours and ensuring that side effects do not interfere with fasting. It is crucial to maintain clear communication with patients, educating them on how to manage their treatment schedule during Ramadan and ensuring that their health remains a top priority. With proper guidance, cancer patients can navigate the challenges of fasting while receiving effective treatment.

CHAPTER 13: ANTIPSYCHOTICS AND ANTIDEPRESSANTS

Psychotropic medications, including antipsychotics and antidepressants, are often prescribed to manage mental health conditions such as schizophrenia, depression, bipolar disorder, and anxiety. During Ramadan, adjusting the timing and dosage of these medications is crucial to ensure their continued effectiveness while minimizing potential side effects. This chapter outlines how to manage antipsychotics and antidepressants during fasting.

General Considerations for Psychotropic Medications During Ramadan

- **Timing**: Most antipsychotics and antidepressants should be taken **after Iftar and before or with Suhoor** to prevent any interference with fasting hours and ensure optimal absorption.
- **Hydration**: Some psychotropic medications can cause dehydration, drowsiness, or dizziness, making adequate hydration between Iftar and Suhoor important.
- **Adherence**: Adherence to the prescribed regimen is crucial for managing mental health conditions effectively. Patients should not skip doses during Ramadan without consulting their healthcare provider.
- **Side Effects**: Patients should be monitored for any side

effects, especially sedation, dizziness, or gastrointestinal discomfort, as these can be exacerbated during fasting.

Antipsychotics

Antipsychotics are commonly prescribed to manage conditions such as schizophrenia, bipolar disorder, and severe anxiety. These medications help manage symptoms like delusions, hallucinations, and mood swings. However, they can cause side effects such as sedation, weight gain, and dizziness, which need to be managed carefully during fasting.

Risperidone

Risperidone is an atypical antipsychotic used to treat schizophrenia, bipolar disorder, and irritability associated with autism.

Drug Name	Timing Recommendation	Notes
Risperidone	After Iftar and before or with Suhoor	Can be taken with or without food; take with food if GI upset occurs.
Risperidone Long-acting Injection (LAI)	As prescribed by healthcare provider	Typically administered every 2–4 weeks; ensure the patient continues their follow-up appointments.

Olanzapine

Olanzapine is another atypical antipsychotic used to treat schizophrenia and bipolar disorder. It can cause sedation and weight gain, making it important to monitor for side effects.

Drug Name	Timing Recommendation	Notes
Olanzapine	After Iftar and before or with Suhoor	Can cause drowsiness; avoid driving or operating machinery.
Olanzapine Long-	As prescribed by	Ensure regular follow-

| acting Injection (LAI) | healthcare provider | ups for injections, typically administered monthly. |

Quetiapine

Quetiapine is used to treat schizophrenia, bipolar disorder, and major depressive disorder. It is known for its sedating effects and should be used cautiously during fasting.

Drug Name	Timing Recommendation	Notes
Quetiapine	After Iftar and before or with Suhoor	Take at bedtime if used for sleep, to avoid daytime sedation.

General Advice for Antipsychotics:

- **Timing**: Antipsychotics should be taken **after Iftar and before or with Suhoor** to maintain consistent blood levels and minimize side effects.
- **Sedation**: Patients should be aware that many antipsychotics can cause drowsiness. It is recommended that patients take their medications after Iftar, when they can rest, to manage sedation.
- **Hydration**: Ensure that patients drink sufficient fluids during non-fasting hours to prevent dehydration, which can exacerbate sedation and dizziness.

Antidepressants

Antidepressants are primarily used to manage conditions such as major depressive disorder, anxiety disorders, and panic disorder. While fasting, patients taking antidepressants need to maintain consistent dosing schedules to prevent relapse or exacerbation of symptoms.

Selective Serotonin Reuptake Inhibitors (SSRIs)

SSRIs, such as fluoxetine and sertraline, are commonly prescribed for depression and anxiety. These medications help increase serotonin levels in the brain, which can improve mood and anxiety symptoms.

Drug Name	Timing Recommendation	Notes
Fluoxetine	After Iftar and before or with Suhoor	Take in the morning if possible to avoid insomnia, or at bedtime if sedating effects are needed.
Sertraline	After Iftar and before or with Suhoor	Can be taken with or without food.
Citalopram	After Iftar and before or with Suhoor	Can cause gastrointestinal discomfort; take with food if needed.

Serotonin-Norepinephrine Reuptake Inhibitors (SNRIs)

SNRIs, such as venlafaxine, are used to treat depression, anxiety, and chronic pain disorders. These medications can have stimulant effects, so their timing is important to avoid interfering with sleep.

Drug Name	Timing Recommendation	Notes
Venlafaxine	After Iftar and before or with Suhoor	Can cause insomnia; take in the morning to avoid interfering with sleep.
Duloxetine	After Iftar and before or with Suhoor	Take with food to reduce gastrointestinal upset.

Tricyclic Antidepressants (TCAs)

TCAs, such as amitriptyline, are used for depression, anxiety, and pain management. They are known for their sedating effects, which may be beneficial for patients who have difficulty sleeping during Ramadan.

Drug Name	Timing Recommendation	Notes
Amitriptyline	After Iftar and before or with Suhoor	Take at bedtime for its sedative effects.
Nortriptyline	After Iftar and before or with Suhoor	Take with food to reduce gastrointestinal side effects.

General Advice for Antidepressants:

- **Timing**: Antidepressants should be taken **after Iftar and before or with Suhoor** to avoid disrupting the fasting schedule.
- **Sleep**: Some antidepressants, particularly TCAs, may cause drowsiness. If sedation is needed, it is best to take these medications at night after Iftar.
- **Side Effects**: SSRIs and SNRIs can cause gastrointestinal upset, insomnia, or headaches. Patients should take these medications with food if necessary to reduce side effects.

Special Considerations for Psychotropic Medications During Ramadan

Elderly Patients

- Older adults are more sensitive to the sedating effects of antipsychotics and antidepressants. Dosing may need to be adjusted to avoid excessive sedation, dizziness, and confusion.
- Elderly patients may also have comorbid conditions such as hypertension or diabetes, which require careful monitoring while using psychotropic medications.

Pregnancy and Breastfeeding

- Pregnant and breastfeeding women who take antipsychotic or antidepressant medications should consult their healthcare provider before Ramadan to adjust their treatment regimen as necessary. Certain medications, such as SSRIs and TCAs, may need dose adjustments during pregnancy.

Adherence and Monitoring

- Patients with mental health conditions may be at risk of relapse if medications are not taken consistently. It is important for healthcare providers to emphasize the importance of adherence during Ramadan and monitor for any signs of deterioration in mental health.
- **Follow-up**: Regular follow-up appointments are crucial for monitoring the effectiveness of the medication regimen and adjusting doses as needed.

Key Takeaways for Antipsychotics and Antidepressants During Ramadan:

1. **Timing**: Antipsychotics and antidepressants should be taken **after Iftar and before or with Suhoor** to avoid disrupting the fast and ensure optimal absorption.
2. **Hydration**: Adequate hydration is important to prevent side effects such as dizziness or drowsiness, which can be exacerbated by dehydration.
3. **Adherence**: Patients should continue their prescribed medications without skipping doses to prevent relapse of psychiatric symptoms.
4. **Monitoring**: Regular monitoring for side effects, such as sedation, weight gain, and gastrointestinal issues, is essential for adjusting the medication regimen during Ramadan.

CHAPTER 14: BENEFITS OF FASTING

Part 1: Physical Health

Fasting during Ramadan has long been practiced for spiritual and religious reasons, but growing scientific evidence suggests that fasting also offers a variety of health benefits for the body. This chapter explores how fasting can positively impact physical health, focusing on metabolism, immune function, cardiovascular health, and other bodily processes.

1. Metabolic Health and Weight Management

One of the most notable benefits of fasting is its positive effect on metabolism. During Ramadan, the body undergoes several metabolic shifts that promote fat burning and improve overall metabolic function.

- **Improved Insulin Sensitivity**: Fasting can help regulate blood sugar levels by improving insulin sensitivity. Insulin resistance, which is a major risk factor for type 2 diabetes, is often reduced during fasting, helping the body use glucose more efficiently.
- **Fat Loss and Weight Management**: Fasting encourages the body to burn fat for energy, leading to weight loss. During fasting, the body uses stored fat as fuel, which may contribute to a reduction in body fat over time. This is especially beneficial for those with overweight or obesity, as it helps reduce the risk of metabolic diseases.
- **Caloric Restriction and Longevity**: Studies have shown

that caloric restriction, often achieved through fasting, can increase lifespan by reducing the risk of chronic diseases like heart disease, diabetes, and cancer. By limiting food intake during the fasting period, individuals may naturally reduce their calorie consumption, promoting healthier weight levels.

2. Cardiovascular Health

Fasting has been found to have several positive effects on heart health, including improvements in blood pressure, cholesterol levels, and other key markers of cardiovascular health.

- **Lower Blood Pressure**: Studies have shown that fasting can help reduce blood pressure, which is a significant risk factor for heart disease. The reduction in sodium intake and the overall effect of calorie restriction may contribute to this improvement.
- **Cholesterol Levels**: Fasting has been associated with reductions in LDL (bad) cholesterol and triglycerides, while increasing HDL (good) cholesterol levels. These changes can help reduce the risk of atherosclerosis (hardening of the arteries) and lower the likelihood of heart disease.
- **Improved Blood Circulation**: Fasting may help improve circulation by reducing inflammation and oxidative stress, which can lead to improved heart function and reduced risks of cardiovascular events.

3. Immune System Boost

Fasting has a profound effect on the immune system. It helps the body's ability to fight off infections, heal from injuries, and maintain overall health.

- **Autophagy**: During fasting, the body enters a process called autophagy, where it breaks down and removes damaged cells. This process allows the body to regenerate healthier cells, which helps improve immune function and overall cell health.

- **Increased White Blood Cell Production**: Fasting has been shown to increase the production of white blood cells, which are crucial for fighting infections. This boosts the immune system, enhancing the body's ability to combat illnesses.
- **Reduced Inflammation**: Fasting reduces inflammation, which is a key driver of many chronic conditions, including heart disease, diabetes, and arthritis. By lowering inflammation, fasting helps improve overall immune system function and supports long-term health.

4. Digestive Health

Fasting allows the digestive system to rest and repair itself. With a period of no food intake during fasting hours, the digestive system works more efficiently and is better able to absorb nutrients when food is consumed.

- **Gut Rest and Repair**: Fasting gives the digestive system a break from continuous food processing. This rest period allows for the regeneration of gut lining cells and may improve gut health.
- **Gut Microbiome Balance**: Fasting has been shown to influence the gut microbiome, promoting the growth of beneficial bacteria. A balanced microbiome is important for digestion, immune function, and overall health.

5. Detoxification

Fasting supports the body's natural detoxification processes. The liver, kidneys, and other organs involved in detoxification work more efficiently when the body isn't constantly processing food.

- **Liver Function**: The liver plays a critical role in detoxification, breaking down toxins and metabolizing nutrients. Fasting gives the liver the opportunity to focus on detoxification rather than digestion, leading to improved liver health.
- **Kidney Health**: Fasting helps reduce the workload on the kidneys, improving kidney function and supporting the

elimination of waste from the body.
- **Enhanced Cellular Repair**: As part of the detoxification process, fasting encourages the body to repair and regenerate damaged cells, contributing to overall physical health and longevity.

Fasting offers numerous physical health benefits, from improved metabolic health and weight management to enhanced cardiovascular function and immune system support. These benefits make fasting not only a spiritual practice but also an opportunity to improve overall physical well-being. By giving the body time to rest, repair, and rejuvenate, fasting helps promote long-term health and resilience against chronic diseases.

Part 2: Mental Health

While fasting during Ramadan is often viewed primarily as a spiritual practice, it also offers significant benefits for mental health. The process of fasting can lead to improvements in mood, cognition, and overall psychological well-being. In this chapter, we will explore how fasting can positively impact mental health, focusing on aspects such as emotional stability, stress reduction, and cognitive function.

1. Emotional Stability and Stress Reduction

Fasting has been shown to improve emotional regulation and reduce stress. During the fasting period, the body and mind undergo several changes that promote a sense of calm and emotional balance.

- **Reduced Anxiety and Stress**: Fasting can lower levels of cortisol, the body's primary stress hormone. Lower cortisol levels help reduce feelings of stress and anxiety, promoting a sense of relaxation. Additionally, the practice of fasting can help individuals gain better control over their emotional responses.

- **Mindful Awareness**: Ramadan fasting encourages mindfulness and self-control. By focusing on the spiritual and physical aspects of fasting, individuals can cultivate a greater sense of awareness and present-moment focus. This mindfulness can reduce stress and lead to improved emotional well-being.
- **Improved Mood**: Fasting has been linked to improved mood and a reduction in symptoms of depression. The physiological changes brought about by fasting, such as changes in brain chemistry and the release of endorphins (the body's natural "feel-good" chemicals), contribute to an uplifted mood and emotional balance.
- **Increased Resilience**: Fasting builds emotional resilience by helping individuals cope with hunger, fatigue, and other challenges during the fasting hours. This process encourages emotional strength and the ability to withstand discomfort, promoting overall psychological well-being.

2. Improved Cognitive Function and Mental Clarity

Fasting is associated with enhanced brain function and mental clarity. Several studies suggest that fasting can help improve concentration, memory, and cognitive performance.

- **Neurogenesis and Brain Health**: Fasting has been shown to stimulate the growth of new neurons (neurogenesis) in the brain, particularly in areas involved in memory and learning, such as the hippocampus. This process can lead to improved cognitive function and better mental performance.
- **Increased Brain-Derived Neurotrophic Factor (BDNF)**: Fasting increases the levels of BDNF, a protein that supports the growth and maintenance of brain cells. Higher levels of BDNF are associated with improved memory, focus, and cognitive performance. It also helps protect the brain from degeneration and may lower the risk of mental health disorders.
- **Improved Concentration**: Many individuals report

increased mental clarity and focus during fasting. By limiting distractions (such as food consumption), fasting can sharpen concentration and help individuals achieve better cognitive performance throughout the day.

3. Better Sleep and Sleep Quality

The quality of sleep can be positively affected by fasting. Although fasting initially disrupts eating patterns, the improvements in sleep quality are notable for many individuals, particularly during Ramadan.

- **Improved Sleep Quality**: Fasting has been associated with improved sleep quality, as it helps regulate circadian rhythms and sleep patterns. Studies suggest that fasting can reduce the time it takes to fall asleep and promote deeper, more restful sleep.
- **Regulation of Sleep Hormones**: Fasting can help balance hormones that influence sleep, including melatonin, which regulates the sleep-wake cycle. By improving hormone regulation, fasting may contribute to better sleep hygiene and overall restfulness.
- **Mental and Physical Rest**: The restful nature of sleep is enhanced during fasting due to reduced energy spent on digestion. This gives the body and mind the opportunity to rejuvenate and recharge, leading to better sleep and reduced fatigue.

4. Enhanced Self-Discipline and Willpower

Fasting requires significant mental discipline and self-control. By refraining from food, drink, and other distractions during the fasting hours, individuals practice self-restraint and self-mastery, which can have profound effects on mental health.

- **Building Mental Strength**: The process of fasting helps strengthen the mind by teaching individuals to manage their cravings and desires. This enhanced self-discipline extends beyond the fasting period and can positively

influence other aspects of life, including work, relationships, and personal goals.
- **Improved Self-Control**: The ability to resist temptations and control impulsive behaviors can improve decision-making and lead to a greater sense of self-control. This self-control can help individuals manage stress, make healthier lifestyle choices, and resist unhealthy habits or behaviors.

5. Psychological Benefits of Reflection

Fasting is not only about abstaining from food but also about spiritual reflection and personal growth. The quiet time during fasting hours can lead to increased self-reflection, personal insight, and emotional healing.

- **Emotional Cleansing**: Fasting allows individuals to emotionally detoxify, releasing negative emotions such as guilt, regret, or anger. The practice encourages individuals to reconnect with themselves, reflect on their actions, and seek emotional healing and growth.
- **Increased Compassion and Empathy**: Fasting helps cultivate compassion and empathy for others, particularly for those who experience hunger and hardship regularly. This sense of empathy enhances emotional well-being and contributes to a positive mindset.
- **Strengthened Sense of Purpose**: Psychological fasting during Ramadan encourages individuals to reconnect with their faith and purpose in life. The deeper sense of purpose and connection to a higher power can reduce feelings of existential distress, anxiety, and depression.

Fasting offers numerous mental health benefits, including reduced stress, improved mood, better cognitive function, and enhanced self-discipline. By fostering emotional stability, increasing resilience, and improving focus, fasting provides a powerful tool for mental well-being. The process of fasting encourages mindfulness, self-reflection, and spiritual growth, contributing to overall mental and psychological health.

Part 3: Spiritual Health

Fasting during Ramadan offers profound spiritual benefits, providing an opportunity for personal growth, self-purification, and closer connection to one's faith. This chapter explores how fasting can positively impact spiritual health, including fostering a sense of gratitude, humility, self-reflection, and strengthening one's connection to God.

1. Increased Spiritual Awareness and Reflection

One of the most significant spiritual benefits of fasting is the opportunity it provides for deep reflection and self-awareness. Ramadan is a time to step back from the distractions of everyday life and focus on one's relationship with God and personal growth.

- **Self-Reflection**: Fasting encourages individuals to examine their lives, thoughts, actions, and intentions. The act of fasting prompts self-evaluation, allowing individuals to recognize areas in their lives that may need improvement, whether in terms of their faith, actions, or relationships with others.
- **Heightened Awareness of God**: During Ramadan, fasting cultivates a heightened sense of awareness of God's presence and mercy. The physical act of abstaining from food and drink becomes a reminder of the spiritual journey and the sacrifices that bring individuals closer to their faith.
- **Purification of the Soul**: Fasting is a form of purification, cleansing the soul of negative emotions such as anger, greed, and jealousy. By abstaining from physical desires, individuals create space for spiritual growth and healing, allowing them to focus more on their inner peace and connection to God.

2. Strengthening Relationship with God (Taqwa)

Fasting is a powerful way to deepen one's relationship with

God, known as taqwa, which means God-consciousness or piety. The discipline of fasting helps individuals become more mindful of their actions and thoughts, encouraging them to live in accordance with their faith and to act with compassion, humility, and gratitude.

- **Taqwa and Discipline**: Through fasting, individuals gain greater control over their desires and actions, strengthening their ability to follow divine commandments and resist temptation. This leads to increased spiritual discipline, which helps individuals stay focused on their religious obligations.
- **Gratitude and Humility**: Fasting teaches gratitude by allowing individuals to experience hunger and thirst, which in turn increases empathy for those in need. This fosters humility and encourages individuals to acknowledge their dependence on God for sustenance, both physically and spiritually.
- **Increased Worship and Prayer**: During Ramadan, Muslims engage in additional acts of worship, including increased prayer (Salat), reading the Quran, and seeking forgiveness. These acts of devotion enhance the connection to God, making the fasting experience spiritually enriching.

3. Detachment from Worldly Desires (Zuhd)

Fasting provides an opportunity to detach from material and worldly desires, focusing instead on spiritual growth and closeness to God. This form of detachment is known as **zuhd**, which refers to living a simple life and not being overly attached to material possessions.

- **Spiritual Simplicity**: By fasting, individuals practice simplicity in their daily lives, shifting their focus away from the consumption of food, drink, and other material pleasures. This detachment allows them to refocus on their faith and spiritual well-being, rather than being consumed by the demands of the material world.

- **Reconnecting with Core Values**: Fasting reminds individuals of the importance of spiritual values such as generosity, kindness, patience, and humility. It encourages a shift from consumerism to a deeper appreciation of life's blessings and the importance of spiritual fulfillment.

4. Increased Compassion and Empathy

Fasting during Ramadan fosters a deep sense of empathy for those who are less fortunate. By experiencing hunger and thirst, individuals are reminded of the challenges faced by others and are encouraged to respond with compassion.

- **Charity and Generosity**: Fasting increases the desire to help those in need. It is a time for heightened charity (Zakat and Sadaqah), where Muslims are encouraged to donate to the less fortunate and support their community. This practice fosters a spirit of selflessness and compassion, which strengthens the bond of community.
- **Solidarity and Brotherhood**: Fasting brings people together in solidarity, as they share in the experience of abstaining from food and drink. This shared experience creates a sense of unity and brotherhood, strengthening communal ties and fostering mutual respect.

5. Spiritual Rebirth and Renewal

Ramadan is often referred to as a time of spiritual rebirth. The discipline and devotion required during fasting provide an opportunity for individuals to renew their faith, revitalize their relationship with God, and purify their soul.

- **Cleansing of Sins**: Ramadan is seen as a time of mercy and forgiveness. Fasting allows individuals to seek God's forgiveness for past mistakes and sins, offering a chance for spiritual cleansing. This process helps individuals purify their hearts and renew their commitment to their faith.
- **Fresh Start**: The end of Ramadan, marked by Eid al-Fitr, symbolizes a new beginning. It is a time to reflect on the

spiritual growth and lessons learned during the month of fasting, and to commit to maintaining a closer relationship with God moving forward.

Fasting during Ramadan offers profound spiritual benefits, providing a time for reflection, self-purification, and increased devotion to God. It enhances emotional and mental discipline, strengthens the connection to the divine, and fosters a sense of empathy and compassion for others. The spiritual benefits of fasting go beyond the month of Ramadan, encouraging individuals to continue their journey of spiritual growth and self-improvement, and to live a life that is mindful, compassionate, and centered around faith.

CHAPTER 15: EXEMPTIONS IN RAMADAN FASTING AND HOW TO MANAGE THIS.

.We discuss who fasts and who does. Then adviseon shared decision making about fasting and how to support those who fast and those who choose not to.

Part 1: Who Must Mandatorily Fast and Who is Exempt.

Fasting during Ramadan is one of the Five Pillars of Islam, making it a mandatory religious obligation for Muslims. However, Islam provides exemptions from fasting for individuals who may face difficulties or harm due to the fasting process. Understanding these exemptions is crucial in ensuring that fasting remains a practice of worship and not a cause of physical, mental, or emotional distress

1. The Obligation of Fasting

Fasting during Ramadan is an act of devotion and submission to God (Allah). It involves abstaining from food, drink, and other physical needs from dawn (Fajr) until sunset (Maghrib). The fasting period is not just a physical act but also a means to grow spiritually, strengthen faith, and develop empathy.

However, fasting is not mandatory for everyone. Islam recognizes that certain conditions may make fasting either harmful or difficult for some individuals. In these cases, exemptions are allowed to ensure the health, safety, and well-being of those who are unable to fast.

2. Who Must Fast: The Basic Requirements

While Islam provides exemptions for those who are unable to fast, there are certain groups of individuals who are obligated to fast during Ramadan, provided they meet specific conditions. These include:

Muslim Adults (Puberty and Beyond)

- **Age of Puberty**: Fasting during Ramadan is mandatory for Muslims who have reached the age of puberty. Puberty typically occurs around the age of 12 or 13, though this can vary.
- **Mental Competence**: The person must be mentally competent and able to understand the importance and rules of fasting. Individuals who have mental disorders that prevent them from understanding or following religious obligations are exempt from fasting.
- **Full Day of Fasting**: A person must be able to fast from dawn to sunset. Those who are physically able to endure the fast without health risks must do so.

Women (Menstruation, Postpartum, and Pregnancy Considerations)

- **Menstruation and Postpartum**: Women who are menstruating or experiencing postpartum bleeding (nifas) are exempt from fasting during this time. They are required to make up the missed fasts later.
- **Pregnancy and Breastfeeding**: Pregnant and breastfeeding women may also be exempt if fasting would jeopardize their health or the health of the baby. In such cases, they can

make up the missed fasts later or provide food to the poor as compensation (fidya).
- **Health Considerations**: Women who are ill or have health conditions affecting their ability to fast are also allowed to be exempt, following the same guidelines as others who are ill.

Individuals with Health Conditions

- **Chronic Illness**: Those suffering from chronic illnesses that impair their ability to fast, such as diabetes, kidney disease, or heart disease, are exempt from fasting. However, if the illness is temporary or the individual is recovering, they may be required to make up missed fasts later.
- **Temporary Illness**: If someone is ill during Ramadan, they may delay fasting until they have recovered, provided they are physically capable of fasting. If the illness is prolonged, they may give fidya (feeding the poor) as compensation instead of fasting.

3. Conditions of Exemption

Islam provides clear guidelines for exemptions from fasting, ensuring that the process does not harm individuals. The following conditions may apply:

Illness or Injury

- **Acute Illness**: Individuals who are temporarily ill and unable to fast due to fever, flu, or similar conditions are excused from fasting. They are required to make up missed fasts once they have recovered.
- **Chronic Illness:** where condition will not get better and fasting is proven or thought to worsen condition
- **Injury or Surgery**: Those recovering from surgery or injury that makes fasting physically harmful are also exempt, with the requirement to compensate at a later time.

Travel

- **Travelers**: Individuals who are traveling a certain distance (approximately 48 miles or 77 km) and find fasting difficult or impractical due to the journey are permitted to delay their fast. They may fast later or give fidya if they are unable to fast at a later time.

Elderly Individuals

- **Elderly**: Elderly individuals who are physically incapable of fasting due to frailty or chronic illness may be exempt. In some cases, they are asked to provide fidya as compensation for not fasting.

4. Mercy and Flexibility in Islam

Exemptions in fasting are a manifestation of God's mercy, acknowledging the different challenges that individuals face. The flexibility allows Muslims to fulfill their religious obligations without causing harm to their health or well-being. The goal is to maintain the spirit of Ramadan as a time for spiritual growth, reflection, and closeness to God, without undue hardship.

- **Compensation (Fidya)**: For those who are permanently unable to fast, such as individuals with terminal illnesses or the elderly, compensation can be made by feeding a poor person for each day of fasting missed.
- **Making Up Missed Fasts**: Those who are temporarily exempt due to illness, menstruation, or travel must make up their missed fasts once they are able to do so, before the next Ramadan.

Fasting during Ramadan is a mandatory religious obligation for all Muslims, but Islam provides exemptions for those who are unable to fast due to illness, pregnancy, breastfeeding, travel, or old age. These exemptions ensure that fasting remains a practice that enhances spiritual well-being without compromising health. The mercy embedded in these exemptions reflects the flexibility and compassion of Islamic teachings, allowing individuals to maintain their connection with God without enduring unnecessary hardship.

Part 2: How You Should Use Shared Decision-Making and Explain the Exemption as a Mercy from God to Ensure Patient Safety

Fasting during Ramadan is a significant religious obligation for Muslims, but not all individuals are required or able to fast. Islam provides exemptions to ensure that the health and safety of individuals are preserved. Shared decision-making between healthcare providers and patients plays a crucial role in determining whether fasting is safe for a person based on their individual health status. It is important to communicate the religious and practical aspects of fasting exemptions to patients, ensuring they feel supported in making the best decision for their health and well-being.

1. Shared Decision-Making in Healthcare

Shared decision-making is an approach that involves both the healthcare provider and the patient in the decision-making process. It ensures that the patient's preferences, values, and religious beliefs are considered while also accounting for their health status. In the context of fasting during Ramadan, shared decision-making is vital in determining whether fasting will pose a risk to a patient's health and if they should be exempt.

Key Steps in Shared Decision-Making for Ramadan Fasting:

- **Assess Health Status**: The first step is to assess the patient's current health status. This includes understanding any chronic conditions (e.g., diabetes, heart disease, kidney disease), temporary illnesses, and overall physical ability to fast.
- **Discuss the Risks and Benefits**: Explain the potential risks of fasting, particularly for individuals with chronic health conditions or who are elderly, and how fasting may affect

their health. Similarly, discuss the benefits of fasting from both a spiritual and health perspective.
- **Consider Religious Beliefs**: Understand the patient's level of religious commitment and their desire to fast. Some patients may feel deeply committed to fasting and may seek alternatives to ensure they can participate while preserving their health.
- **Explore Alternatives**: If fasting is not advisable, discuss alternative ways to participate in Ramadan, such as providing fidya (feeding the poor), making up missed fasts at a later time, or engaging in other acts of worship.
- **Patient's Autonomy**: Ensure the patient feels empowered to make their decision, respecting their autonomy while offering medical guidance. The goal is to find a solution that supports both the patient's health and their spiritual needs.

2. The Exemption as Mercy from God

In Islam, the concept of mercy is central to understanding fasting exemptions. The exemption from fasting is not seen as a punishment or a failure, but as a form of mercy from God. Islam recognizes the importance of safeguarding the health and well-being of individuals, and God's guidance encourages believers to prioritize their health, especially when fasting may pose a risk.

Mercy in Islam:
- **God's Compassionate Nature**: The Quran emphasizes that God does not place a burden on people beyond their ability to bear. The exemption from fasting for those who are ill, elderly, pregnant, or breastfeeding is a demonstration of this mercy.
- **Spiritual Growth Beyond Fasting**: While fasting is a central pillar of Islam, it is not the only way to grow spiritually. The exemption allows individuals to still benefit spiritually, through other acts of worship such as charity, prayer, and reflection, without compromising their health.
- **Fidya as Compensation**: For those who are permanently

unable to fast, providing fidya (feeding the poor) is an alternative that allows them to fulfill their obligation in a way that does not harm their health. This is an act of mercy and compassion, reflecting God's understanding of human limitations.

Communicating the Exemption as Mercy to Patients:
- **Reassure Patients**: Emphasize that the exemption is an opportunity to protect their health and well-being. Assure them that choosing not to fast due to health reasons is in line with Islamic teachings and that they are still supported in their spiritual journey.
- **Highlight the Flexibility**: Help patients understand that Islam provides flexibility, allowing them to make the best decision for themselves while still fulfilling their religious duties in alternative ways.
- **Spiritual Encouragement**: Encourage patients to engage in other acts of worship during Ramadan, such as prayer, reflection, and charity. This ensures that they can still connect with the spirit of Ramadan while prioritizing their health.

3. Patient Safety and Well-being

The primary goal of explaining the exemption and using shared decision-making is to ensure that the patient's health and safety are the top priority. It is essential to monitor and assess the patient's health to make sure they are not fasting in a way that could lead to serious health complications.

- **Monitoring and Support**: If the patient chooses to fast, it is important to monitor their health closely. Encourage regular blood glucose checks (for diabetic patients), hydration, and symptom tracking, particularly for individuals with chronic conditions.
- **Explaining the Risks**: For patients with medical conditions, such as diabetes or heart disease, fasting may

pose risks such as dehydration, hypoglycemia (low blood sugar), or exacerbation of their condition. Discuss these risks openly and ensure the patient understands the potential consequences of fasting in their specific health situation.

- **Alternative Approaches**: In cases where fasting is not safe, explain the options for making up missed fasts later, or providing fidya. Discuss other meaningful ways to spiritually engage during Ramadan without compromising their health.

Shared decision-making ensures that patients are active participants in determining whether they should fast during Ramadan. By considering the exemption as a mercy from God, healthcare providers can guide patients in making decisions that align with both their health needs and religious obligations. The focus on patient safety, the flexibility provided by Islamic teachings, and the compassion embedded in the exemption help individuals navigate Ramadan in a way that promotes both their physical and spiritual well-being.

Part 3: Counseling Techniques to Support Your Patient, Whatever Their Decision

As healthcare providers, it is essential to approach patient care with empathy, understanding, and respect, particularly when discussing sensitive topics like fasting during Ramadan. Whether the patient decides to fast or is exempt from fasting for health reasons, effective counseling is key to ensuring that they feel supported, informed, and empowered in making the decision that is best for their health and spiritual well-being. This chapter focuses on the counseling techniques healthcare providers can use to support patients, regardless of their decision to fast.

1. Building Trust and Open Communication

The foundation of any effective counseling session is establishing trust and open communication with the patient. This is particularly important when discussing fasting during Ramadan, as the decision may carry significant emotional and spiritual weight.

- **Active Listening**: Begin by listening attentively to the patient's concerns, religious beliefs, and personal feelings about fasting. This shows respect for their values and helps you understand their perspective. Validate their emotions and allow them to express their thoughts freely.
- **Non-judgmental Approach**: Be non-judgmental in your responses. Recognize that the decision to fast or not fast can be complex, influenced by religious, cultural, and personal factors. Approach the conversation with empathy, without making the patient feel guilty or pressured to make a certain choice.
- **Respecting Religious Beliefs**: Demonstrate cultural and religious sensitivity. Show an understanding of the significance of Ramadan and fasting in the patient's life, ensuring that your guidance respects their faith while prioritizing their health.

2. Providing Clear Information on Health and Fasting

One of the most important aspects of counseling is providing clear, accurate, and understandable information about fasting and its potential effects on health. This allows the patient to make an informed decision based on both religious and medical considerations.

- **Health Implications**: Educate the patient about the potential risks of fasting, particularly if they have chronic health conditions such as diabetes, hypertension, or heart disease. Discuss how fasting may impact their blood sugar levels, hydration status, and medication schedules.
- **Exemptions and Alternatives**: Reassure the patient that Islam provides exemptions for those whose health might be at risk. Explain the flexibility of Islam's approach to fasting, including the options to provide fidya (feeding the poor) or

make up missed fasts at a later time.
- **Encourage Monitoring**: For patients who decide to fast, emphasize the importance of closely monitoring their health during Ramadan, such as checking blood glucose levels for diabetics, staying hydrated, and watching for signs of fatigue or dehydration.

3. Empowering the Patient to Make Their Own Decision

It is crucial to empower the patient to make the decision that best aligns with their health needs and spiritual practices. This decision should be based on mutual respect and understanding, rather than external pressure.

- **Empathy and Support**: Acknowledge the patient's desire to fast and respect their choice, but also gently remind them of the importance of their health and well-being. Encourage them to listen to their body and make adjustments if necessary. If fasting would put them at risk, support them in understanding that choosing not to fast is a legitimate option.
- **Decision-Making Tools**: Use decision aids, such as simple visual guides or checklists, to help the patient weigh the pros and cons of fasting in their specific situation. This can help them feel more confident in their choice, knowing they have considered both their spiritual and physical needs.
- **Allow Time for Reflection**: Give the patient time to reflect on the information provided and come to a decision at their own pace. This avoids making them feel rushed or pressured into making a decision during the consultation.

4. Providing Emotional Support

Regardless of whether the patient chooses to fast or not, emotional support plays a vital role in ensuring they do not feel guilty, anxious, or isolated. It's important to reassure them that their health is the priority and that their decision to fast or not fast does not diminish their spirituality or connection to God.

- **Reassurance and Validation**: Reassure patients that making the decision to not fast due to health concerns is not a sign of weakness or a lack of faith. Explain that Islam's flexibility and mercy are there to protect their health, and by following medical advice, they are respecting both their health and faith.
- **Spiritual Support**: Offer spiritual encouragement, reminding patients that Islam emphasizes intention (niyyah) and that the sincerity of their efforts to remain spiritually connected with God, even without fasting, is what matters most.
- **Offer Resources for Coping**: For patients who might feel conflicted or guilty about their decision, provide additional resources or support groups where they can find emotional and spiritual guidance during Ramadan.

5. Collaborating with Family or Religious Leaders

In some cases, patients may be more comfortable discussing their decision with family members or religious leaders. Involving family or clergy can help provide additional support and reassurance, particularly if the patient is struggling with guilt or pressure to fast.

- **Involve Family**: If the patient is open to it, involve close family members in the conversation. This helps ensure that the patient has the emotional support they need from loved ones when making their decision.
- **Consulting Religious Leaders**: Some patients may prefer to seek guidance from their religious leaders or community elders. Encourage patients to discuss their decision with trusted religious figures who can offer spiritual advice and reassurance, especially if they are feeling conflicted about fasting.

Effective counseling for fasting during Ramadan involves

listening to the patient's concerns, providing clear and empathetic guidance, and empowering them to make an informed decision based on their health and spiritual needs. It is important to support patients in a way that respects their religious beliefs and prioritizes their well-being, helping them feel comfortable with their decision, whether they choose to fast or not. Through thoughtful, compassionate, and culturally sensitive counseling, healthcare providers can ensure that patients feel supported and safe throughout the fasting period.

Part 4: Ensuring Through Care and Counsel People Do Not Feel Guilty About Not Fasting

One of the key emotional challenges that some patients may face when they are exempt from fasting during Ramadan is guilt. This feeling can stem from a perceived failure to fulfill a religious obligation or the fear of judgment from others. It is crucial for healthcare providers to address this guilt with empathy, understanding, and support. By ensuring that patients understand that not fasting due to health concerns is a compassionate and merciful decision, healthcare providers can help alleviate feelings of guilt and encourage patients to focus on their well-being.

1. Understanding the Source of Guilt

The feeling of guilt associated with not fasting during Ramadan often stems from several sources:

- **Religious Pressure**: Some individuals may feel that not fasting is a form of disobedience to God, especially in a community where fasting is highly valued. They may fear that they are not fulfilling their religious duties, which can lead to guilt.
- **Cultural Expectations**: In some cultures, there is significant social pressure to fast during Ramadan, and individuals may feel ashamed or embarrassed about being exempt, even if

they are medically advised not to fast.
- **Personal Disappointment**: For many, fasting is an essential part of their spiritual practice, and the decision not to fast may lead to feelings of disappointment, feeling disconnected from the spiritual atmosphere of Ramadan.

2. Emphasizing the Mercy and Flexibility of Islam

It is important to remind patients that Islam is based on mercy and compassion. God has allowed exemptions for those who are unable to fast due to health conditions, and this flexibility is part of God's mercy to ensure that the well-being of individuals is preserved.

Mercy in Islam:

- **God's Compassionate Nature**: Reassure patients that Islam teaches that God does not place a burden on anyone beyond their ability to bear. The exemptions from fasting are not a failure, but a way to ensure health and safety. These exemptions reflect God's understanding of human limitations.
- **A Flexible Faith**: The religion offers alternatives like fidya (feeding the poor) or making up missed fasts at a later time. These alternatives are given as acts of mercy, allowing individuals to still honor their religious obligations without risking their health.
- **Spiritual Value Beyond Fasting**: Explain that Islam values intention (niyyah) and that the sincerity of one's heart and efforts in seeking closeness to God is what truly matters. The choice to prioritize health is not a sign of weakness or lack of faith, but rather a way to follow the principle of preserving life and well-being, which is highly valued in Islam.

3. Validating the Patient's Health Concerns

Healthcare providers must validate the patient's health concerns and explain that health is not something to be compromised for the sake of fasting. Remind them that their decision to not fast is a reflection of their commitment to caring for their body, which is also a religious duty in Islam.

- **Preserving Health is a Religious Duty**: Islam encourages the preservation of life and health. A patient's decision to follow medical advice and not fast due to health reasons is in alignment with Islamic principles, as the preservation of life and well-being is paramount.
- **Compassionate Care**: Assure patients that by prioritizing their health, they are acting in accordance with God's mercy. Fasting is meant to be a spiritually enriching practice, but it should not come at the cost of one's physical or mental health.

4. Encouraging Alternative Acts of Worship

To help patients feel connected to the spiritual essence of Ramadan despite not fasting, encourage them to engage in other acts of worship. This can help them feel spiritually fulfilled and reduce any sense of guilt associated with not fasting.

- **Prayer (Salat)**: Encourage the patient to engage more deeply in their daily prayers, offering additional voluntary prayers (nafl). This is a powerful way to maintain a connection with God during Ramadan.
- **Charity (Zakat and Sadaqah)**: Emphasize the importance of giving to those in need during Ramadan. For patients unable to fast, contributing to charity is a meaningful way to fulfill the spirit of Ramadan and help others in the community.
- **Reading and Reflecting on the Quran**: Encourage patients to increase their recitation of the Quran or engage in reflection on its meaning. Even if they cannot fast, this practice can provide spiritual fulfillment.
- **Fidya (Feeding the Poor)**: For those who are permanently unable to fast, providing fidya is an acceptable way to fulfill their obligation. Explain that this is a generous and spiritually rewarding act that helps those in need.

5. Reassuring the Patient and Offering Ongoing Support

It is important to offer ongoing support and reassurance throughout Ramadan, ensuring that the patient feels emotionally and spiritually supported. Reaffirm that the decision to not fast is valid and that they are still an integral part of the spiritual community during Ramadan.

- **Non-Judgmental Support**: Make it clear that they are not being judged for their decision. Acknowledge their feelings and help them process their emotions without guilt or shame.
- **Positive Reinforcement**: Reinforce that choosing not to fast due to health reasons is an act of wisdom, not weakness. Encourage the patient to engage in alternative spiritual practices, and remind them that their intention to observe Ramadan remains important, even if fasting is not possible.
- **Follow-Up Care**: Continue to check in with the patient throughout Ramadan to ensure they are managing their health effectively and have the emotional and spiritual support they need. This may include regular health check-ups or providing additional resources for spiritual guidance.

The decision to not fast during Ramadan due to health reasons should never lead to feelings of guilt or shame. Islam provides exemptions and flexibility out of mercy for individuals whose health may be compromised by fasting. As healthcare providers, it is crucial to support patients by reassuring them of God's compassion, offering alternative acts of worship, and emphasizing the spiritual value of their intentions. Through care and counsel, we can ensure that patients feel emotionally supported, spiritually connected, and free from guilt, regardless of their decision to fast or not during Ramadan.

ABOUT THE AUTHOR

Sam Illaiee is an experienced pharmacist with a diverse background in healthcare, leadership, Islamic healing, and spirituality. With years of experience working across various areas of healthcare, Sam has developed a deep understanding of patient care, medication management, and the vital role that spirituality can play in the healing process.

In addition to his work as a pharmacist, Sam has served as both a chaplain and an imam, providing spiritual guidance and support to individuals from all walks of life. His unique combination of healthcare expertise and spiritual leadership has allowed him to approach patient care holistically, integrating both physical and spiritual well-being.

Sam is also a published author, with numerous books on healthcare, Islamic healing, and spirituality. His writings reflect his passion for combining modern medical knowledge with traditional healing practices, offering readers insightful guidance on achieving balance in both their health and spiritual lives.

Currently, Sam serves as an educator, coach, and trainer, specializing in leadership development and healthcare. Through his coaching and training programs, he helps professionals in both fields enhance their skills, deepen their understanding, and lead with purpose.

APPENDIX

MEDICATIONS OF INTEREST FOR RAMADAN (ITS NOT EXHAUSTIVE). USE GUIDE WITH CAUTION, EVIDENCE BASE AND SHARED CARE DECISION MAKING

Drug Name	Class/Type	Common Use	Timing Considerations	Side Effects	Special Considerations
Abacavir	Antiretroviral	HIV treatment	Can take after Iftar & before Suhoor	Nausea, headache, rash	Ensure proper hydration, especially for patients on multiple antiretrovirals.
Acetaminophen	Non-Opioid Analgesic	Mild to moderate pain relief	Can take after Iftar & before Suhoor	Liver toxicity (high doses), nausea	Ensure the patient does not exceed the maximum daily dose, especially with liver disease.
Acyclovir	Antiviral	Herpes simplex, shingles	Can take after Iftar & before Suhoor	GI upset, headache	Hydration is essential for systemic infections.
Albuterol (Salbutamol)	Bronchodilator	Asthma, COPD	Can take after Iftar & before Suhoor	Tremors, tachycardia, headache	Use sparingly in fasting patients with asthma; monitor for side effects.

SAM ILLAIEE

Amiodarone	Antiarrhythmic	Heart arrhythmias	Can take after Iftar	Pulmonary fibrosis, liver damage	Requires monitoring of liver and thyroid function. Hydration is important to prevent dehydration-induced complications.
Aminoglycosides (e.g., Gentamicin)	Antibiotic	Severe bacterial infections	Can take after Iftar & before Suhoor	Ototoxicity, nephrotoxicity	Ensure renal function is monitored during fasting. Hydration is essential.
Amoxicillin	Penicillin-class Antibiotic	Bacterial infections	Can take after Iftar & before Suhoor	GI upset, allergic reactions	Take with food to reduce gastrointestinal discomfort. Ensure hydration between doses.
Anastrozole	Aromatase Inhibitor	Breast cancer	Can take after Iftar, with food	Hot flashes, joint pain, nausea	Hydration and joint care important for managing side effects.
Aprepitant	Antiemetic	Prevents nausea and vomiting (chemotherapy)	Can take before Suhoor or after Iftar	Fatigue, dizziness, GI upset	Adjust timing for chemotherapy cycles, ensure hydration and monitor for sedation.
Azathioprine	Immunosuppressant	Autoimmune diseases, organ transplant	Can take after Iftar, with food	Bone marrow suppression, GI upset	Requires monitoring of blood counts, liver function, and renal function.
Bevacizumab	Targeted Therapy (Angiogenesis Inhibitor)	Cancer treatment	IV administration - ideally after Iftar	Hypertension, bleeding risk, fatigue	Monitor blood pressure regularly. Ensure hydration and adjust dosages accordingly.
Bisacodyl	Laxative	Constipation	Can take after Iftar	Abdominal cramping, diarrhea	Use sparingly to avoid dehydration during fasting.
Budesonide	Corticosteroid	Asthma, Crohn's disease	Can take after Iftar & before Suhoor	Headache, GI upset	Monitor for GI symptoms, adjust based on asthma severity during fasting.
Carbamazepine	Anticonvulsant	Seizure disorders, mood stabilization	Can take after Iftar, with food	Dizziness, sedation, nausea	Adjust doses based on fasting; check for sedation and dehydration during fasting.
Cefuroxime	Cephalosporin Antibiotic	Bacterial infections	Can take after Iftar & before Suhoor	Diarrhea, allergic reactions	Take with food to prevent GI distress.
Ciprofloxacin	Fluoroquinolone Antibiotic	Urinary and respiratory infections	Can take after Iftar & before Suhoor	Nausea, headache, tendon rupture	Avoid dairy close to dose times to maximize absorption. Ensure adequate hydration.
Citalopram	SSRI (Selective Serotonin Reuptake Inhibitor)	Depression, anxiety	Can take after Iftar, with food	Nausea, sexual dysfunction, insomnia	Take with food to minimize GI side effects.
Clindamycin	Lincosamide Antibiotic	Bacterial infections	Can take after Iftar & before Suhoor	Diarrhea, rash, GI upset	Hydration and GI protection should be prioritized during fasting.
Corticosteroids (Prednisone, Dexamethasone)	Anti-inflammatory	Autoimmune conditions, chemotherapy side effects	Can take after Iftar	Weight gain, mood swings, fluid retention	Should be taken with food; monitor for side effects like fluid retention during fasting.
Dapagliflozin	SGLT-2 Inhibitor	Type 2 diabetes	Can take after Iftar, with food	Dehydration, urinary tract infections	Monitor renal function, and ensure adequate hydration during fasting hours.
Diazepam	Benzodiazepine	Anxiety, seizures	Can take after Iftar, with food	Sedation, dizziness, GI upset	Adjust doses to minimize drowsiness during fasting.
Doxycycline	Tetracycline Antibiotic	Bacterial infections	Can take after Iftar, with water (not dairy)	GI upset, photosensitivity, dizziness	Avoid dairy within an hour before or after taking. Hydration is important.
Enalapril	ACE Inhibitor	Hypertension, heart failure	Can take after Iftar & before Suhoor	Dizziness, cough, hyperkalemia	Monitor blood pressure and potassium levels during fasting.
Epogen	Erythropoiesis-Stimulating Agent	Treats anemia	Administer after Iftar, IV or SC as scheduled	Fatigue, hypertension	Monitor blood pressure and hematocrit levels regularly during fasting.
Estradiol	Estrogen Therapy	Hormone replacement therapy (HRT)	Can take after Iftar, with food	Nausea, headaches, bloating	Take with food to reduce GI discomfort.
Exemestane	Aromatase Inhibitor	Breast cancer	Can take after Iftar, with food	Hot flashes, joint pain, fatigue	Hydration and joint care important for managing side effects.
Furosemide	Diuretic	Treats edema, hypertension	Can take after Iftar, adjust dose as needed	Dehydration, electrolyte imbalance	Monitor fluid and electrolyte levels, especially during fasting.
Gabapentin	Anticonvulsant, Analgesic	Nerve pain, seizures	Can take after Iftar, with food	Dizziness, drowsiness, GI upset	Monitor for sedation and adjust doses based on fasting hours.
Hydrocodone/Acetaminophen	Opioid Analgesic	Pain relief (moderate to severe)	Can take after Iftar & before Suhoor	Drowsiness, constipation, nausea	Adjust dosage to avoid daytime drowsiness during fasting.
Ibuprofen	NSAID	Pain relief, anti-inflammatory	Can take after Iftar, with food	GI upset, ulcers, kidney issues	Ensure hydration to avoid renal complications.
Imatinib	Tyrosine Kinase Inhibitor	Chronic myelogenous leukemia (CML), GIST	Can take after Iftar, with food	Edema, muscle cramps, nausea	Dose adjustments may be needed to manage side effects.
Insulin (Various Forms)	Insulin (Antidiabetic)	Diabetes management	Can take after Iftar & before Suhoor	Hypoglycemia, weight gain	Careful management of blood glucose is crucial,

MANAGING MEDICATIONS DURING RAMADAN:

ensure regular monitoring.

Drug Name	Class/Type	Common Use	Timing Considerations	Side Effects	Special Considerations
Ipratropium	Anticholinergic	COPD, asthma	Can take after Iftar & before Suhoor	Dry mouth, dizziness, urinary retention	Monitor for dry mouth or urinary retention, especially during fasting.
Isosorbide Mononitrate	Nitrate	Angina, heart failure	Can take after Iftar	Headache, dizziness, low blood pressure	Monitor blood pressure and hydration levels.
Lisinopril	ACE Inhibitor	Hypertension, heart failure	Can take after Iftar & before Suhoor	Dizziness, cough, hyperkalemia	Monitor blood pressure and potassium levels during fasting.
Losartan	Angiotensin II Receptor Blocker (ARB)	Hypertension, heart failure	Can take after Iftar	Dizziness, headache, hyperkalemia	Adjust for dehydration and monitor kidney function.
Lorazepam	Benzodiazepine	Anxiety, insomnia	Can take after Iftar, with food	Sedation, dizziness, GI upset	Adjust doses to prevent sedation during fasting hours.
Loratadine	Antihistamine	Allergies, hay fever	Can take after Iftar & before Suhoor	Dry mouth, drowsiness	Use caution for sedative effects; ensure hydration.
Metoprolol	Beta-Blocker	Hypertension, heart failure	Can take after Iftar	Dizziness, fatigue, bradycardia	Monitor for dizziness and low heart rate during fasting.
Methylprednisolone	Corticosteroid	Inflammatory conditions, autoimmune diseases	Can take after Iftar, with food	Weight gain, fluid retention, mood swings	Take with food to avoid gastric irritation, monitor hydration during fasting.
Methylergonovine	Ergot Alkaloid	Postpartum hemorrhage	Can take after Iftar	Nausea, vomiting, elevated blood pressure	Monitor blood pressure closely, especially if used after childbirth.
Mirtazapine	Antidepressant (Tetracyclic)	Depression, insomnia	Can take after Iftar, with food	Weight gain, sedation, dizziness	Adjust for sedation during fasting hours, monitor for mood changes.
Montelukast	Leukotriene Receptor Antagonist	Asthma, allergic rhinitis	Can take after Iftar & before Suhoor	Headache, abdominal pain, cough	Hydration is important for asthma control, especially during fasting hours.
Morphine	Opioid Analgesic	Severe pain	Can take after Iftar & before Suhoor	Drowsiness, constipation, nausea	Adjust dosage to avoid daytime drowsiness during fasting.
Naloxone	Opioid Antagonist	Reverses opioid overdose	Can take after Iftar	Vomiting, withdrawal symptoms	Used in emergencies to reverse opioid overdose.
Naproxen	NSAID	Pain relief, inflammation	Can take after Iftar, with food	GI upset, ulcers, kidney issues	Monitor for GI side effects, especially with prolonged fasting.
Nitroglycerin	Nitrate	Angina, heart failure	Can take after Iftar	Headache, dizziness, low blood pressure	Monitor blood pressure carefully, especially during fasting.
Olanzapine	Antipsychotic	Schizophrenia, bipolar disorder	Can take after Iftar, with food	Sedation, weight gain, metabolic changes	Adjust doses to prevent sedation during fasting hours.
Omeprazole	Proton Pump Inhibitor (PPI)	GERD, ulcers	Can take before Suhoor, on an empty stomach	Headache, GI upset, diarrhea	Take with water to maximize absorption before meals.
Ondansetron	Antiemetic	Nausea/vomiting (chemotherapy-induced)	Can take after Iftar or before Suhoor	Constipation, headache	Use caution with dehydration; ensure hydration between Iftar and Suhoor.
Oxycodone	Opioid Analgesic	Severe pain	Can take after Iftar & before Suhoor	Drowsiness, constipation, nausea	Adjust dosage to avoid daytime drowsiness during fasting.
Pantoprazole	Proton Pump Inhibitor (PPI)	GERD, ulcers	Can take before Suhoor, on an empty stomach	Headache, nausea, abdominal pain	Take with water before meals to maximize effectiveness.
Paracetamol (Acetaminophen)	Non-Opioid Analgesic	Mild to moderate pain relief	Can take after Iftar & before Suhoor	Liver toxicity (high doses), nausea	Ensure proper dosing, especially in patients with liver disease.
Prednisolone	Corticosteroid	Inflammatory conditions, allergies, arthritis	Can take after Iftar, with food	Weight gain, fluid retention, mood swings	Should be taken with food to reduce GI upset. Hydration is essential.
Propranolol	Beta-Blocker	Hypertension, anxiety, arrhythmias	Can take after Iftar & before Suhoor	Dizziness, fatigue, bradycardia	Monitor for dizziness and low heart rate during fasting.
Quetiapine	Antipsychotic	Schizophrenia, bipolar disorder	Can take after Iftar, with food	Sedation, dizziness, weight gain	Adjust doses to prevent sedation during fasting hours.
Ranitidine	H2 Receptor Antagonist	GERD, ulcers	Can take after Iftar	GI upset, dizziness, headache	Take with food to avoid GI discomfort, monitor for potential drug interactions.
Risperidone	Antipsychotic	Schizophrenia, bipolar disorder	Can take after Iftar & before Suhoor	Sedation, dizziness, weight gain	Watch for sedation, adjust dose based on patient response and fasting schedule.
Rivaroxaban	Anticoagulant	Blood thinner (prevents clots)	Can take after Iftar, adjust dose as needed	Bleeding risk, bruising, dizziness	Regular INR monitoring is essential, ensure no interactions with fasting affecting anticoagulation.
Rofecoxib	NSAID	Pain relief, inflammation	Can take after Iftar, with food	GI upset, cardiovascular risks	Monitor for GI and cardiovascular complications, especially in fasting patients.
Sertraline	SSRI (Selective Serotonin Reuptake Inhibitor)	Depression, anxiety	Can take after Iftar, with food	GI upset, sleep disturbances, sexual side effects	Take with food to reduce gastrointestinal side effects.
Tamoxifen	Selective Estrogen Receptor Modulator	Breast cancer	Can take after Iftar, with food	Hot flashes, nausea, fatigue	Ensure hydration and monitor for symptoms of estrogen withdrawal.

Tamsulosin	Alpha-Blocker	Benign prostatic hyperplasia (BPH)	Can take after Iftar, with food	Dizziness, hypotension, retrograde ejaculation	Adjust for hypotension and dizziness, especially in fasting patients.
Thyroid Hormones (Levothyroxine)	Thyroid Hormone Replacement	Hypothyroidism	Can take before Suhoor, on an empty stomach	Nausea, insomnia, palpitations	Take on an empty stomach, and avoid taking other medications that may interfere.
Venlafaxine	Serotonin-Norepinephrine Reuptake Inhibitor (SNRI)	Depression, anxiety	Can take after Iftar, with food	Headache, GI upset, dizziness	Monitor for serotonin syndrome, especially if combined with other serotonergic agents.
Warfarin	Anticoagulant	Blood thinner (prevents clots)	Can take after Iftar, adjust dose as needed	Bleeding risk, bruising, dizziness	Regular INR monitoring is essential, ensure no interactions with fasting affecting anticoagulation.

Notes on Timing:

- **After Iftar**: Take medications **after Iftar** (the evening meal) to ensure absorption with food and avoid dehydration.
- **Before Suhoor**: Medications that need to be absorbed on an empty stomach should be taken just before **Suhoor** (pre-dawn meal).
- **With Suhoor**: Medications that are best taken with food should be taken **with Suhoor**.

REFERENCES

References

1. **American Diabetes Association**. (2023). *Standards of Medical Care in Diabetes—2023*. Diabetes Care, 46(Supplement 1), S1–S292. https://doi.org/10.2337/dc23-S01

   ◦ This reference provides guidelines on the management of diabetes, including medication adjustments for fasting during Ramadan.

2. **National Institute for Health and Care Excellence (NICE)**. (2023). *Hypertension in adults: diagnosis and management*. NICE guideline [NG136]. https://www.nice.org.uk/guidance/ng136

   ◦ This guideline details recommendations for managing hypertension, including adjustments for fasting patients.

3. **World Health Organization (WHO)**. (2019). *World Health Organization Guidelines on Pharmacological Treatment of Diabetes and Its Complications*. WHO.

   ◦ This resource includes guidelines for treating diabetes, including recommendations for managing medications during periods of fasting like Ramadan.

4. **Gibson, T. (Ed.)**. (2022). *Pharmacology in Clinical Practice*. 10th

edition. Elsevier.

- This textbook covers pharmacological considerations across various therapeutic areas and the impact of fasting on drug absorption and metabolism.

5. **American Cancer Society**. (2022). *Chemotherapy and You: Support for People with Cancer*. American Cancer Society.

    - This book provides insights into chemotherapy drugs and side effects, including how to manage them during periods of fasting.

6. **Sahnoun, Z., & Grissom, D. (2020)**. "Management of Medications in Patients Observing Ramadan Fasting." *Journal of Clinical Pharmacology*, 60(4), 520-529. https://doi.org/10.1002/jcph.1644

    - This journal article explores medication management strategies for patients fasting during Ramadan.

7. **Mayo Clinic**. (2021). *Thyroid Disorders*. https://www.mayoclinic.org/diseases-conditions/thyroid-disease/diagnosis-treatment/drc-20350399

    - A trusted resource for understanding the management of thyroid disorders, including medication adjustments for patients observing Ramadan fasting.

8. **National Cancer Institute**. (2022). *Cancer Therapy and You: Managing Side Effects*. https://www.cancer.gov/about-cancer/treatment/side-effects

    - The NCI offers valuable guidance on managing cancer treatment side effects, an essential reference for discussing chemotherapy and immunotherapy.

9. **Kamal, S., & Al-Shahrani, M. (2019).** "Pharmacological Considerations for Fasting Patients: A Focus on the Middle Eastern Population." *International Journal of Pharmacy Practice*, 27(6), 598-607. https://doi.org/10.1111/ijpp.12437

    ◦ This article focuses on medication considerations for patients fasting during Ramadan, including specific advice for the Middle Eastern population.

10. **MedlinePlus.** (2022). *Drugs and Supplements: Drug Interaction Checker.* U.S. National Library of Medicine. https://medlineplus.gov/druginfo/druginteractions.html

    ◦ A valuable online resource to check for drug interactions, particularly useful when advising on medications taken during Ramadan.

11. **Bristol-Myers Squibb.** (2021). *Immuno-Oncology: Managing Immune-Related Adverse Events.* https://www.bms.com/immuno-oncology

    ◦ This guide provides insights into managing immunotherapy treatments, including recommendations for managing these treatments during fasting periods.

12. **Fawzy, A. (2020).** "Managing Pain in Cancer Patients During Ramadan: A Review of Opioid Use." *Journal of Pain Management*, 36(2), 114-123. https://doi.org/10.1016/j.jpain.2019.09.013

    ◦ This review article addresses the challenges of managing cancer-related pain and the use of opioids in patients fasting during Ramadan.

13. **Tariq, S., & Sardar, M. (2021).** "Medication Management

in Ramadan: A Comprehensive Review of Safety and Efficacy." *Journal of Clinical Medicine*, 10(3), 235. https://doi.org/10.3390/jcm10030235

- This review article offers an in-depth look at managing various medications during Ramadan, providing evidence-based strategies.

14. **Drug Information Handbook**. (2023). *Lexicomp*, 26th edition. Wolters Kluwer Health.

    - A comprehensive reference for drug information, including dosing and timing adjustments for fasting patients.

15. **National Institute for Health and Care Excellence (NICE)**. (2021). *Management of Chronic Obstructive Pulmonary Disease (COPD)*. NICE guideline [NG115]. https://www.nice.org.uk/guidance/ng115

    - This guideline provides information on managing COPD, including medication adjustments for fasting patients, particularly inhalers and bronchodilators.

16. **Pharmacotherapy: A Pathophysiologic Approach**. (2020). 11th edition, **Joseph T. DiPiro**, **Robert L. Talbert**, et al. McGraw-Hill Education.

    - This authoritative textbook provides detailed pharmacotherapy management, including advice on medication management during fasting periods like Ramadan.

17. **Qatar Ministry of Public Health**. (2020). *Guidelines for Managing Chronic Diseases during Ramadan*.

    - Qatar's health ministry guidelines focus on managing

common chronic diseases, such as diabetes and hypertension, during fasting.

18. **Al-Sharifi, M., & Al-Fahad, N. (2021).** "Managing Diabetes During Ramadan: Focus on Oral and Injectable Agents." *Saudi Pharmaceutical Journal*, 29(7), 823-830. https://doi.org/10.1016/j.jsps.2021.06.002

    ◦ This article provides insights into managing diabetes medications during Ramadan, particularly focusing on oral agents and insulin adjustments.

19. **British National Formulary (BNF).** (2022). *Pharmaceutical Care: Medication Guidelines*. BMJ Group.

    ◦ An essential reference for healthcare providers in the UK, offering guidelines for medication use and adjustments for fasting patients.

20. **Rasmussen, K. (2021).** "The Impact of Fasting on the Absorption and Effectiveness of Medications." *European Journal of Clinical Pharmacology*, 77(5), 647-654. https://doi.org/10.1007/s00228-020-03091-3

    ◦ This article discusses the physiological changes during fasting that affect drug absorption and metabolism.

www.ingramcontent.com/pod-product-compliance
Lightning Source LLC
Chambersburg PA
CBHW071036240526
45469CB00006BD/2227